Absolute Obstetric Anesthesia Review

Cassandra Wasson · Albert Kelly
David Ninan · Quy Tran

Absolute Obstetric Anesthesia Review

The Complete Study Guide for
Certification and Recertification

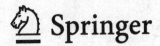 Springer

Cassandra Wasson
Riverside University Health System -
Medical Center
Moreno Valley, CA
USA

Albert Kelly
Riverside University Health System -
Medical Center
Moreno Valley, CA
USA

David Ninan
Riverside University Health System -
Medical Center
Loma Linda, CA
USA

Quy Tran
Harbor–UCLA Medical Center
Torrance, CA
USA

ISBN 978-3-319-96979-4   ISBN 978-3-319-96980-0   (eBook)
https://doi.org/10.1007/978-3-319-96980-0

Library of Congress Control Number: 2018957090

This Springer imprint is published by the registered company Springer Nature Switzerland AG
The registered company address is: Gewerbestrasse 11, 6330 Cham, Switzerland

This book is dedicated to the Riverside University Health System Anesthesia Program and my classmates of the anesthesia class of 2019 (Tyler Gouvea, Kellie Morris, Devangi Patel, and Ngoc Truong). Without the love and support of my attendings, classmates, and staff at RUHS, this book would not be possible.

Preface

The field of anesthesiology is ever expanding and the need for subspecializing is becoming more and more common in order to provide the best care for the most complex patients and improve patient safety and outcomes. With an increased number of high-risk patients (such as those congenital heart disease) becoming pregnant, the need for anesthesiologists subspecializing in obstetrics is growing.

Although the number of fellowships available for obstetric anesthesia is increasing, the number of invaluable resources available to these trainees is not. *Absolute Obstetric Anesthesia Review* was created to provide a concise, easy to follow outline of obstetric anesthesia for anesthesiology residents, obstetric anesthesiology fellows, and any anesthesiologist providing care to obstetric patients. It is written to follow the outline set forth by the American Board of Anesthesiology (ABA) to be an invaluable resource for in-service exam and board exams. It goes to a fellow-level depth of information. It provides testable information for the boards, as well as practical tips for clinical practice.

We hope you find this book helpful, easy to use, and a quick read. It is small enough to carry during your obstetric anesthesia rotation, rather than the larger textbooks that are over 1000 pages in length. We hope the concise nature of this book allows you to cover more material in your limited time to study, allowing you more time for the clinical aspects of obstetric anesthesia.

Moreno Valley, CA, USA

Loma Linda, CA, USA
Torrance, CA, USA

Cassandra Wasson
Albert Kelly
David Ninan
Quy Tran

Contents

Part I
Maternal Physiology

Effects of Pregnancy on Uptake and Distribution

1. MAC for volatiles is decreased up to 40% in pregnancy
   (a) Rate of induction is faster due to greater minute ventilation and reduced functional residual capacity (FRC)
2. Pregnant women have a larger volume of distribution due to expanded extracellular volume and total body water, so recovery from many anesthetic drugs is faster
3. The potency of some medications is increased due to decreased levels of albumin and alpha 1-acid glycoprotein for drug binding leading to more unbound drug concentration in plasma

C. Wasson et al., *Absolute Obstetric Anesthesia Review*, https://doi.org/10.1007/978-3-319-96980-0_1

Respiratory

Chapters 2, 16, and 17 Chestnut's

1. Airway: increased edema, vascularity, and capillary engorgement of the larynx and the nasal and oropharyngeal mucosa.
   (a) Nasal breathing can be difficult
   (b) Prone to epistaxis; avoid nasal intubation if possible
   (c) Anticipate difficult oral intubation
   (d) Smaller endotracheal tubes should be used
2. Respiratory changes during pregnancy compared to pre-pregnancy values:
   (a) No change: FEV_1, FVC, FEV_1/FVC, peak expiratory flow, flow-volume loop, closing capacity, pulmonary compliance, and diffusing capacity
   (b) Decreased: pulmonary resistance and chest wall compliance
      (i) Chest wall compliance is decreased because the ligamentous attachments of the ribs are relaxed and the AP and transverse diameters of the thoracic cage are increased due to the hormone relaxin
      (ii) Total pulmonary and airway resistances decrease due to hormonal relaxation of tracheobronchial tree smooth muscles
   (c) Increased: Diaphragm excursion (due to its higher resting position)
3. Respiratory physiology changes during pregnancy
   (a) Increased: Dead space (+45%); inspiratory reserve volume (+5%); minute ventilation (+45%); alveolar ventilation (+45%); tidal volume (TV) (+45%); and inspiratory capacity (+15%)
      (i) TV increases due to a decrease in expiratory reserve volume
      (ii) Minute ventilation is increased due to an increase in tidal volume rather than respiratory rate
         1. Progesterone increases the sensitivity of the respiratory center to CO_2 leading to the increased minute ventilation

(b) Decreased: expiratory reserve volume (−25%); residual volume (−15%); FRC (−20%); and total lung capacity (−5%)

    (i) FRC decreases due to the uterus expanding resulting in reduction of ERV and RV

        1. O_2 reserve decreases and causes the potential for airway closure and atelectasis

(c) Unchanged: respiratory rate and vital capacity

4. Pregnancy frequently causes respiratory alkalosis with a compensatory metabolic acidosis

    (a) The normal $PaCO_2$ during pregnancy is 30 mmHg

    (b) Normal blood gas during pregnancy: pH 7.44, PaCO2 30–34 mmHg, HCO_3 20–22 mEq/L, PaO_2 105 mmHg.

    (c) Clinical implication: Maternal hyperventilation due to labor pain or anxiety may cause fetal acidosis because further reduction in $PaCO_2$ can lead to decreased uteroplacental perfusion and a left shift of the maternal oxygen dissociation curve

5. O_2 consumption is increased

6. Changes during labor (mitigated by neuraxial anesthesia):

    (a) Increased minute ventilation causes $PaCO_2$ levels as low as 10–15 mmHg

    (b) Increased O_2 consumption due to the increased metabolic demands of hyperventilation, uterine activity, and maternal expulsive efforts during the second stage of labor, which leads to anaerobic metabolism and increased lactate concentrations

Cardiovascular

3

Chapters 2, 16 and 17 Chestnut's

1. EKG changes common during pregnancy: shortened PR and QT intervals; axis shift (to the right during the first trimester and to the left during the third trimester); depressed ST segments; and low-voltage T waves
2. Echocardiography changes common during pregnancy: increase in end diastolic volume of both left and right ventricles. Slight increase in mitral and tricuspid annuluses causing regurgitations. Eccentric hypertrophy of left ventricle
3. Hemodynamics observed during pregnancy
   (a) Increased: cardiac output (+50%); stroke volume (+25%); heart rate (+25%); left ventricular end-diastolic volume; ejection fraction (EF)
   (b) Decreased: systemic vascular resistance (SVR) (−20%)
   (c) Unchanged: left ventricular end-systolic volume; left ventricular stroke work index; pulmonary capillary wedge pressure; pulmonary artery diastolic pressure; central venous pressure
4. The greater blood volume of pregnancy causes cardiac eccentric hypertrophy
5. S1 is accentuated and S2 splitting is exaggerated
6. S3 is not pathologic during pregnancy
7. Systolic ejection murmur (grade II) is common during pregnancy due to augmented blood flow from increased intravascular volume
   (a) Diastolic murmurs are abnormal
8. MAP decreases with pregnancy

© Springer Nature Switzerland AG 2019
C. Wasson et al., *Absolute Obstetric Anesthesia Review*,
https://doi.org/10.1007/978-3-319-96980-0_3

9. Cardiac output is highest in the immediate postpartum period
   (a) Due to relief of vena caval compression, contractions of the uterus (auto-transfusion of blood into systemic circulation), decreased lower extremity venous pressure, and reduced maternal vascular capacitance
   (b) Cardiac output returns to prepregnancy levels between 12 and 24 weeks postpartum
10. Aortocaval compression occurs after 18–20 weeks' gestation
   (a) Important to left tilt to maintain cardiac pre-load

Renal

Chapter 2 Chestnut's

1. Kidneys enlarge by as much as 30%
2. Collecting system dilates; hydronephrosis is very common
3. Creatinine clearance increases and BUN decreases due to an increase in GFR and renal plasma flow during pregnancy
   (a) Normal Cr level during pregnancy is 0.5–0.6 mg/dL
   (b) Normal BUN level during pregnancy is 8–9 mg/dL
4. Urinary protein, albumin, and glucose excretion are increased during pregnancy

© Springer Nature Switzerland AG 2019
C. Wasson et al., *Absolute Obstetric Anesthesia Review*,
https://doi.org/10.1007/978-3-319-96980-0_4

Liver

1. Liver size, morphology, and blood flow do not change
2. Bilirubin, ALT, AST, and lactic dehydrogenase are upper limits of normal during pregnancy
3. ALP increases 2–4× due to production from placenta
4. Increased risk of gallbladder disease during pregnancy due to the inhibitory effects of progesterone on GI smooth muscles, leading to gallbladder hypomotility and subsequent biliary stasis

C. Wasson et al., *Absolute Obstetric Anesthesia Review*,
https://doi.org/10.1007/978-3-319-96980-0_5

Gastrointestinal

1. Pregnancy compromises the integrity of the lower esophageal sphincter (LES), alters the anatomic relationship of the esophagus to the diaphragm and stomach, and raises intragastric pressure
   (a) Stomach is displaced upward toward the left side of the diaphragm
   (b) Decreased LES tone is likely due to smooth muscle relaxation properties of progesterone
   (c) Changes return to pre-pregnancy levels by 48 h post-partum
2. High rate of GERD during pregnancy. Risk factors include gestational age, GERD prior to pregnancy, and multiparity
   (a) Maternal age has an inverse correlation
3. Gastric acid pH and volume is unchanged in pregnancy
4. Rate of gastric emptying is unchanged during pregnancy, but significantly prolonged during labor
   (a) Esophageal peristalsis and intestinal transit are slowed

© Springer Nature Switzerland AG 2019
C. Wasson et al., *Absolute Obstetric Anesthesia Review*,
https://doi.org/10.1007/978-3-319-96980-0_6

Hematology

1. RBC volume increases (~30%), but plasma volume increases more (~55%), leading to a dilutional anemia "physiologic anemia of pregnancy" (normal hemoglobin is 11.6 g/dL, hematocrit 35.5%)
   (a) Plasma volume increases due to increased renin activity due to higher estrogen levels, which enhances renal sodium and water absorption
2. Lower hematocrit decreases blood viscosity and lowers resistance to blood flow, which is essential to maintain the patency of the uteroplacental vascular bed.
3. Total blood volume increases (~45%), which allows delivery of nutrients to the fetus, protects the mother from hypotension, and decreases the risks associated with hemorrhage at delivery
4. Total plasma protein and albumin concentrations both decrease in pregnancy
5. Globulin levels increase, so albumin/globulin ratio decreases
6. Plasma cholinesterase concentrations decrease in pregnancy
7. Benign leukocytosis is common in pregnancy (WBC can rise to ~13,000/mm^3 during labor)
8. Changes in coagulation and fibrinolytic parameters at term:
   (a) Increased fibrinogen (a.k.a. factor I), factors VII, VIII, IX, X, and XII
   (b) Decreased factor XI and XIII
   (c) Factors II and V are unchanged
   (d) PT and PTT are shortened
   (e) Platelet count and function are changed, but bleeding time is unchanged
9. Enhanced platelet turnover, clotting, and fibrinolysis
   (a) Normal D-dimer in pregnancy can be as high as 500–1700 ng/mL compared to <500 ng/ml in nonpregnant adults

© Springer Nature Switzerland AG 2019
C. Wasson et al., *Absolute Obstetric Anesthesia Review*,
https://doi.org/10.1007/978-3-319-96980-0_7

1. The placenta is the fetal "lung" and has a fifth of the O$_2$ transfer efficiency of the adult lung
2. Placenta provides ~8 mL O$_2$/min/kg fetal body weight
3. Delivery of oxygen to the fetus is predominantly flow limited (i.e., maternal delivery of blood to the uterus controls fetal oxygen transfer)
4. O$_2$ transfer across the placenta depends on the O$_2$ partial pressure gradient between maternal blood and fetal blood
   (a) O$_2$ dissolved in plasma diffuses across the villous membranes and O$_2$ bound to hemoglobin (Hgb) is released and diffuses across the placenta
5. Factors favoring fetal oxygen uptake:
   (a) Oxygen affinity: Fetal oxyhemoglobin (Hb F) dissociation curve is shifted left (high oxygen affinity; P50: 19 mmHg) and maternal (Hb A) dissociation curve is shifted right (P50: 27 mmHg), allowing greater O$_2$ transfer to fetus
   (b) Oxygen-carrying capacity: The hemoglobin concentration of fetal blood is high 15 g/dL compared with the mother's 12 g/dL
6. Bohr effect also enhances O$_2$ transfer to fetus; fetal-maternal transfer of CO$_2$ makes maternal blood more acidotic and fetal blood more alkalotic causing a shift in maternal and fetal oxyhemoglobin dissociation curves favoring unloading of maternal oxygen to fetus

© Springer Nature Switzerland AG 2019
C. Wasson et al., *Absolute Obstetric Anesthesia Review*,
https://doi.org/10.1007/978-3-319-96980-0_8

Placental CO_2 Exchange

1. Transferred as dissolved CO_2, carbonic acid, bicarbonate ion (predominant form), carbonate ion, and carbaminohemoglobin
2. CO_2 is 20× more diffusible than O_2 and readily crosses the placenta
3. Only dissolved CO_2 crosses the placenta. Carbonic anhydrase in RBCs convert bicarbonate ion to CO_2.
4. CO_2 transfer is augmented by the Haldane effect (higher affinity for CO_2 in maternal deoxyhemoglobin than fetal oxyhemoglobin)

© Springer Nature Switzerland AG 2019
C. Wasson et al., *Absolute Obstetric Anesthesia Review*,
https://doi.org/10.1007/978-3-319-96980-0_9

Placental Blood Flow

1. Major determinant of oxygen and nutrient delivery to the fetus
2. Preeclampsia and intrauterine growth restriction (IUGR) are associated with chronic placental insufficiency
3. Blood supply to the uterus is mainly from the uterine arteries (branch of the anterior division of the internal iliac artery) and to a less extent the ovarian arteries (branches off abdominal aorta)
4. Venous drainage of the uterus occurs via the uterine veins to the internal iliac veins and the ovarian veins to the inferior vena cava on the left and the renal vein on the right
5. Uterine blood flow increases during pregnancy from 50 to 100 mL/min prior to pregnancy to 700–900 mL/min at term
6. Uterine blood flow exceeds the minimum required to satisfy fetal O_2 demand, causing a margin of safety
   (a) Uteroplacental blood flow can decrease by 50% for limited periods before fetal hypoxia and metabolic acidosis occurs
7. Uteroplacental circulation is a maximally dilated, low-resistance system without autoregulation (i.e., perfusion is pressure dependent)
8. Placental perfusion decreases during contractions
   (a) Inversely related to strength of contraction and rise in intrauterine pressure
9. Uterine blood flow = (uterine perfusion pressure)/(uterine vascular resistance)
   (a) Uterine perfusion pressure = uterine arterial pressure – uterine venous pressure

© Springer Nature Switzerland AG 2019
C. Wasson et al., *Absolute Obstetric Anesthesia Review*,
https://doi.org/10.1007/978-3-319-96980-0_10

10. Causes of decreased uterine blood flow:
    (a) Decreased perfusion pressure
        (i) Decreased uterine arterial pressure (supine position (aortocaval compression); hemorrhage/hypovolemia; drug-induced hypotension; hypotension during sympathetic blockade)
        (ii) Increased uterine venous pressure (vena caval compression; uterine contractions; drug-induced uterine hypertonus (oxytocin, local anesthetics); skeletal muscle hypertonus (seizures, Valsalva maneuver))
    (b) Increased uterine vascular resistance
        (i) Endogenous vasoconstrictors (catecholamines (stress) and vasopressin (released during hypovolemia))
        (ii) Exogenous vasoconstrictors (epinephrine; vasopressors (phenylephrine>ephedrine); and high concentrations of local anesthetics
11. Pregnancy causes a decreased response to endogenous and exogenous vasoconstrictors due to increased levels of progesterone, prostacyclins, and nitric oxide.
12. Although Angiotensin II levels are increased 2–3× during pregnancy, it has little effect on uterine vascular resistance.
13. Infusion of angiotensin II has minimal effect on uteroplacental blood flow while increasing systemic blood pressure.
14. In contrast to angiotensin II, alpha-adrenergic agonists affect uterine circulation more than systemic circulation
15. Angiotensin II affects systemic vascular resistance with little effect on uterine vascular resistance causing an increase in uterine blood flow
16. Neuraxial anesthesia may increase or decrease uterine blood flow
    (a) Decreased due to induced hypotension
    (b) Increased uterine blood flow due to pain relief, decreased sympathetic activity, and decreased maternal hyperventilation
        (i) Hyperventilation causes vasoconstriction and may decrease uterine blood flow
17. Agents commonly used to induce general anesthesia have minimal or no direct adverse effect on uteroplacental blood flow.
    (a) Uteroplacental perfusion may be affected indirectly by changes in blood pressure and sympathetic response to laryngoscopy and endotracheal intubation
18. Magnesium decreases uterine vascular resistance and increases uterine blood flow

Barrier Function

1. The placenta is an imperfect barrier (allows many substances to cross)
2. Cytochrome P-450 isoenzymes are located in the placenta, and some may be inducible
   (a) These enzymes may metabolize agents and decrease fetal exposure
3. Placenta may also bind substances to minimize fetal exposure to and accumulation of substances

© Springer Nature Switzerland AG 2019
C. Wasson et al., *Absolute Obstetric Anesthesia Review*,
https://doi.org/10.1007/978-3-319-96980-0_11

Part II

Maternal-Fetal Considerations

Pharmacology of Local Anesthetic Drugs

12

1. All local anesthetics (except cocaine) contain a desaturated carbon ring and a tertiary amine connected by an alkyl chain.
   (a) The alkyl chain (ester vs. amide linkage) determines whether it is an amino-ester or amino-amide.
   (b) All local anesthetic are weak bases because the tertiary amine portion acts as a proton acceptor.
2. Amino-amides (e.g., lidocaine, bupivacaine, ropivacaine) undergo hepatic microsomal metabolism
3. Amino-esters (e.g., chloroprocaine, cocaine, tetracaine) are hydrolyzed by pseudocholinesterase
4. When pH > pKa, more drug is ionized
   (a) Un-ionized form is lipid soluble and diffuses through the cell membrane
   (b) Ionized form is more active in blocking the Na^+ channel
5. Mechanism of action of local anesthetics: interference with sodium-ion conductance
6. 2-Chloroprocaine
   (a) Hydrolyzed rapidly by plasma pseudocholinesterase
   (b) Half-life: 11–21 s in plasma; 1.5–6.4 min epidural
7. Lidocaine
   (a) Half-life ~114 min epidural
   (b) Metabolized to two active compounds (glycinexylidide (GX) and monoehylglycinexylidide (MEGX))
   (c) Predominately bound to alpha-1-acid glycoprotein (AAG) in plasma. Pregnancy has decreased AAG, causing an increased free plasma fraction of lidocaine in pregnant women
8. Bupivacaine
   (a) Half-life: 12–13 h plasma
   (b) Highly binds to both AAG and albumin (96%).

© Springer Nature Switzerland AG 2019
C. Wasson et al., *Absolute Obstetric Anesthesia Review*,
https://doi.org/10.1007/978-3-319-96980-0_12

9. Ropivacaine
   (a) Shorter half-life than bupivacaine (~5 h vs 12)
   (b) Highly binds to albumin and AAG (92%)
10. H2 blockers (especially cimetidine) bind to cytochrome P-450, reducing hepatic blood flow and renal clearance of local anesthetics
11. Pre-eclampsia decreases clearance of local anesthetics due to reduced hepatic blood flow, abnormal liver function, and decreased intravascular volume
12. Local anesthetic toxicity signs/symptoms (earliest to latest) (affects CNS before the CV system): numbness of tongue/lightheadedness/tinnitus, muscular twitching, unconsciousness, convulsions, coma, respiratory arrest, cardiovascular depression
    (a) Convulsions are due to selective blockade of CNS inhibitory neurons, causing CNS excitation
    (b) CNS depression/coma occurs due to reversible blockade of both inhibitory and excitatory pathways
13. Local anesthetic CNS toxicity risk (greatest to least): bupivacaine > ropivacaine > levobupivacaine > lidocaine > 2-chloroprocaine. Tetracaine, etidocaine, and mepivacaine are rarely used in obstetric anesthetic practice
14. Treatment of local anesthetic systemic toxicity (LAST):
    (a) Mild cases: discontinue drug, administer supplemental O2, maintain normal ventilation
    (b) If signs of CNS excitation, small dose of thiopental (50 mg) or diazepam (2.5–5 mg) or midazolam (1–2 mg) may prevent convulsions
    (c) If active convulsions, maintain oxygenation and ventilation to prevent hypoxemia, hypercarbia, and acidosis (as these may worsen local anesthetic toxicity)
       (i) Intubate if necessary
       (ii) Terminate convulsions with small dose of thiopental or diazepam
       (iii) Maintain maternal circulation with left uterine displacement and vasopressor as needed
    (d) Treat cardiac arrest according to ACLS guidelines
    (e) 20% Lipid emulsion therapy may be necessary for refractory cardiac arrest due to local anesthetic toxicity
       (i) Bolus 1.5 ml/kg (lean body mass) IV over 1 min. Repeat bolus once or twice for persistent cardiovascular collapse
       (ii) Continue infusion at 0.25 mg/kg/min, and double to 0.5 ml/kg/min if blood pressure remains low.
       (iii) Continue infusion for at least 10 min after cardiovascular stability is achieved
    (f) Avoid vasopressin, calcium channel blockers, beta-adrenergic blockers, and local anesthetics.
       (i) Amiodarone is first line for arrhythmias
    (g) Reduce epinephrine doses to <1 ug/kg.
    (h) Arrangement for cardiopulmonary bypass (CPB) for persistent cardiovascular instability. CPB may be necessary while waiting for local anesthetic to diffuse from cardiac receptors.

15. Tissue Toxicity
    (a) Rare. Due to direct neural trauma, infection, injection of toxic dose of local anesthetic, or the injection of the wrong drug
    (b) Cauda equina syndrome, sacral nerve root deficits, or transient neurologic toxicity can occur after subarachnoid injection of lidocaine
    (c) Neurotoxicity of local anesthetics is concentration dependent
    (d) Transient neurologic symptoms (TNS) is dyesthesia or low back pain radiating to the buttocks, thighs, or calves that occurs after spinal anesthesia.
        (i) Associated with lidocaine, and lithotomy position
        (ii) Pregnancy may reduce the incidence of TNS
16. Allergic reactions
    (a) True allergy to local anesthetic is rare
    (b) Anaphylactic and anaphylactoid reactions may be due to additives in local anesthetic (e.g. methylparaben and meta-bisulfite)
    (c) Allergy: urticarial, bronchospasm, facial edema, and/or cardiovascular collapse
    (d) Pharmacologic management:
        (i) Inhibition of mediator synthesis and release
        (ii) Reversal of the effects of the mediators on target organs
        (iii) Prevention of recruitment of other inflammatory processes
        (iv) Drugs used: catecholamines (epinephrine (mainstay), norepinephrine, or isoproterenol), phosphodiesterase inhibitors, antihistamines (diphenhydramine), and corticosteroids (hydrocortisone or methylprednisone).

Pharmacology of Local Anesthetic Adjuvants

13

1. Opioids
   (a) Neuraxial opioids cause analgesia without loss of sensation or proprioception
   (b) 3 classifications:
      (i) Naturally occurring (e.g. morphine, codeine, papaverine)
      (ii) Semisynthetic (e.g. heroin, hydromorphone, oxymorphone, hydrocodone, oxycodone, buprenorphine, nalbuphine)
      (iii) Synthetic (e.g. meperidine, fentanyl, sufentanil, alfentanil, and remifentanil)
         1. Meperidine is unique in that it possesses weak local anesthetic properties
   (c) Produce analgesia by binding to G protein-coupled opioid receptors, which inhibits both adenylate cyclase and voltage-gated calcium channels, causing inhibition of release of excitatory afferent neurotransmitters (e.g. glutamate, substance P, and other tachykinins)
   (d) Parenteral opioids affect both spinal and supraspinal
   (e) Neuraxial opioids bind presynaptic and postsynaptic receptor sites located at substantia gelatinoa (rexed lamina II) in dorsal horn of spinal cord to block transmission of pain-related information
   (f) Four opioid receptors
      (i) Mu – analgesia, miosis, bradycardia, sedation, respiratory depression, decreased GI transit
      (ii) Kappa – analgesia, sedation, respiratory depression, diuresis, psychotomimesis
      (iii) Delta – analgesia
      (iv) Nociception/orphanin receptor – pain processing in spinal and supraspinal areas
   (g) Onset and duration of analgesia and side effects of neuraxial opioid administration depend on the type of opioid receptor that is activated, the dose, lipid solubility, and rate of movement and clearance of the opioid in the cerebral spinal fluid (CSF)

© Springer Nature Switzerland AG 2019
C. Wasson et al., *Absolute Obstetric Anesthesia Review*,
https://doi.org/10.1007/978-3-319-96980-0_13

(h) Side effects of neuraxial opioids: fewer side effects with more lipid-soluble opioids
  (i) Sensory changes
    1. Patients feel like they cannot breathe or swallow
    2. Motor function is not impaired, so reassure patient that symptoms will subside in 30–60 min
  (ii) Nausea and vomiting
    1. Multiple factors, such as pregnancy, physiology of labor itself, pain associated with labor, or parenteral administration of opioid prior to neuraxial opioids
    2. Treatments: Metoclopramide, ondansetron, scopolamine, cyclizine, or dexamethasone
  (iii) Pruritus
    1. Most common side effect of neuraxial opioids
    2. More common intrathecal than with epidural administration.
    3. Decreased incidence and severity with lower dose of opioid or co-administration of local anesthetic
    4. Morphine may cause pruritus by stimulating 5-HT3 receptors
      (a) Patients who receive 5-HT3 receptor antagonists (e.g. ondansetron) had less pruritus and less severity of pruritus
    5. Other treatments of pruritus: IV naloxone (40–80 mcg) or diphenhydramine (25 mg) or nalbuphine (2.5–5 mg IV)
      (a) Nalbuphine less likely to reverse neuraxial opioid analgesia
      (b) Opioid-induced pruritus is unrelated to histamine release, however, diphenhydramine is still used for its sedative effect
  (iv) Hypotension
    1. Due to pain relief and decreased maternal levels of catecholamines
    2. May be due to sympathetic blockade if local anesthetic administered intrathecally with opioid
  (v) Respiratory depression
    1. Risk factors:
      (a) Drug and its pharmacokinetics
      (b) Drug dose
      (c) Concomitant CNS depressants
    2. Rare, but potentially lethal, complication. ASA practice guidelines recommend monitoring all patients who received neuraxial opioids for ventilation (e.g. respiratory rate, etCO2), oxygenation (e.g. pulse oximetry) and level of consciousness
      (a) For lipophilic opioid: monitor continuously for 20 min after injection, followed by at least Q1 h for 2 h.
      (b) For hydrophilic opioid: Monitor at least Q1 h for the first 12 h, and then at least Q2 h for the next 12 h.
  (vi) Urinary retention
  (vii) Delayed gastric emptying

1. Greatest with parenteral, followed by intrathecal, and then epidural opioids.

    (viii) Recrudescence of oral HSV infections

2. Epinephrine
    (a) Added to epidural and spinal local anesthetic to increase duration of anesthesia, reduce peak plasma drug concentrations, improve block reliability, and intensify analgesia/anesthesia
    (b) Systemic absorption may increase maternal heart rate (HR) and may transiently decrease uterine activity as a result of beta-adrenergic stimulation
    (c) More effective at prolonging duration of local anesthetic with high intrinsic vasodilatory property (e.g. lidocaine)
    (d) Does not prolong bupivacaine or ropivacaine as these local anesthetics have inherent vasoconstricting properties.
    (e) Epinephrine has analgesic effects produced by stimulation of alpha2-adrenergic receptors

3. Bicarbonate
    (a) Adding bicarbonate to local anesthetic increases pH closer to pKa, which increases proportion of drug in un-ionized form, increasing amount available to penetrate nerve sheath and membrane
    (b) Quickens onset of analgesia, intensifies anesthesia, and improves spread to sacral dermatomes
    (c) May cause precipitation (greatest with bupivacaine)
    (d) Increases risk of hypotension

4. Alpha2-adrenergic agonists (e.g. clonidine)
    (a) Provides analgesia without affecting sensation or producing motor blockade
    (b) Potentiates the quality and duration of epidural analgesia
    (c) Produces hypotension by acting on alpha2-adrenergic receptors on preganglionic cholinergic neurons causing sympatho-inhibition at spinal cord and brain.
    (d) Produces sedation by alpha2-adrenergic stimulation in locus ceruleus
    (e) NOT recommended in US for use in obstetric analgesia due to risk of maternal hypotension and bradycardia and abnormal FHR tracings

5. Neostigmine
    (a) Prevents breakdown of acetylcholine in the spinal cord, which allows it to bind to nicotinic and muscarinic receptors in the dorsal horn. Stimulation of muscarinic receptors causes release of GABA in dorsal horn leading to analgesia
    (b) More effective at alleviating somatic pain than visceral pain therefore limited efficacy for labor pain when used as sole agent.
    (c) Intrathecal neostigmine causes severe nausea unresponsive to standard antiemetics
    (d) Not routinely used in OB anesthesia, and its neuraxial use is not FDA approved

Pharmacology of Oxytocic Drugs

14

1. Oxytocin
   (a) Indications: labor arrest during the active phase of the 1st stage of labor and prophylaxis and treatment of uterine atony
      (i) For postpartum uterine atony, diluted IV solution at infusion rate of 20–80 units/h) or 10 units IM
   (b) Oxytocin has an antidiuretic effect, which may cause water intoxication with seizures and even coma
   (c) Uterine hyperstimulation may occur and interrupt uterine blood flow
      (i) Fetus may become hypoxemic and fetal compromise may result
   (d) Bolus administration of oxytocin causes peripheral vasodilation, which may cause hypotension and reflex tachycardia
2. Methylergonovine is an ergot alkaloid
   (a) Indicated for uterine atony refractory to oxytocin
   (b) Given 0.2 mg IM
   (c) Side effects: vasoconstriction, severe HTN (sometimes resulting in cardiovascular accident (CVA) and seizures), elevated pulmonary artery pressure, and pulmonary edema
   (d) May also cause coronary artery vasoconstriction and have been associated with myocardial ischemia or infarction
   (e) Relative contraindications: HTN, preeclampsia, peripheral vascular disease, and ischemic heart disease
3. Prostaglandin E1 (i.e., Misoprostol (cytotec))
   (a) Indications: refractory uterine atony
   (b) Given 800–1000 mg per rectum (PR)
   (c) Side effects: malaise, fever, chills, diarrhea, nausea, and vomiting, hyperthermia

© Springer Nature Switzerland AG 2019
C. Wasson et al., *Absolute Obstetric Anesthesia Review*,
https://doi.org/10.1007/978-3-319-96980-0_14

4. 15-methyl prostaglandin $F_{2\alpha}$ (carboprost, hemabate)
   (a) Indications: refractory uterine atony
   (b) Give 250 ug IM when other drugs have failed
   (c) May be repeated at 15- to 90-min intervals up to a maximum of 8 doses
   (d) Side effects: malaise, fever, chills, diarrhea, nausea, and vomiting
   (e) May cause bronchospasm and pulmonary vasoconstriction, so caution in asthmatics and pulmonary HTN

Mechanisms of Placental Transfer, Placental Transfer of Specific Drugs

15

1. Most drugs cross the placenta
   (a) Large, organic ions do not (e.g. insulin and heparin)
   (b) All anticonvulsants cross the placenta
2. Factors influencing transfer:
   (a) Physiochemical characteristics of the drug:
      (i) Molecular size: compounds <500 Da cross placenta easily
      (ii) Uncharged molecules pass easily
      (iii) Protein binding decreases transfer
      (iv) Lipid soluble agents cross easily
      (v) Degree of ionization
         1. Un-ionized molecules are more lipid soluble
         2. Acidotic fetus has larger proportion of ionized drug, causing "ion trapping"
   (b) Concentration of free drug in maternal blood. Affected by:
      (i) Dose
         1. Higher doses cause higher maternal blood concentration
      (i) Site of administration
         2. Rate of absorption and peak plasma concentration depends on vascularity of site of administration
         3. Local anesthetic absorption greatest to least (BICEPSS): Blood > intercostal > caudal > epidural > plexus (brachial) > spinal/sciatic/femoral > subcutaneous
      (ii) Metabolism and excretion
      (iii) Effects of adjuvants (e.g. epinephrine)
   (c) Permeability of the placenta
   (d) Hemodynamic events occurring within the fetal-maternal unit

3. Drugs that cross the placenta:
   (a) Anticholinergic agents (atropine and scopolamine)
   (b) Neostigmine
   (c) Antihypertensive agents (beta-adrenergic receptor antagonists, nitroprusside, and nitroglycerin)
   (d) Benzodiazepines (diazepam and midazolam)
   (e) All anticonvulsants
   (f) Induction agents (propofol and thiopental)
   (g) Inhalational anesthetics (halothane, isoflurane, sevoflurane, desflurane, and nitrous oxide)
   (h) Local anesthetics
   (i) Opioids
   (j) Vasopressors (ephedrine)
4. Drugs that don't cross the placenta:
   (a) Glycopyrrolate
   (b) Antioagulants and reversal (heparin, low molecular weight heparin, protamine)
   (c) Muscle relaxants (both depolarizing (succinylcholine) and non-depolarizing)
   (d) Sugammadex
   (e) Insulin

Fetal Disposition of Drugs

16

1. Fetal tissue uptake of local anesthetics influenced by:
   (a) Fetal plasma protein binding
   (b) Lipid solubility
   (c) Degree of ionization of the drug
   (d) Hemodynamic changes that affect the distribution of fetal cardiac output
       (i) Increased blood flow to vital organs (e.g. heart, brain, adrenal glands) during asphyxia
2. Intrathecal lipophilic opioids may cause fetal bradycardia
   (a) Possibly due to decreased circulating maternal catecholamines associated with rapid onset of analgesia
       (i) Decreasing epinephrine (which has a tocolytic effect via beta-2 receptor agonism) may increase uterine tone, leading to decreased uteroplacental perfusion and fetal hypoxia since uteroplacental perfusion occurs during uterine relaxation
   (b) Fetal heart rate changes are usually transient and may be managed successfully with conservative measures:
       (i) Supplemental O2
       (ii) Position changes to relieve aortocaval compression
       (iii) Vasopressor therapy to treat hypotension
       (iv) Discontinuation of oxytocin infusion
       (v) Administration of tocolytic agent for persistent uterine hypertonus (e.g., nitroglycerin)
3. Anticonvulsants
   (a) Increased risk of congenital anomalies, especially cleft lip with or without cleft palate, congenital heart disease, and digital malformations
   (b) Valproic acid or carbamazepine increases risk of neural tube defects and other malformations

© Springer Nature Switzerland AG 2019
C. Wasson et al., *Absolute Obstetric Anesthesia Review*,
https://doi.org/10.1007/978-3-319-96980-0_16

    (c) Fetal hydantoin syndrome (in newborns exposed to phenytoin): Craniofacial abnormalities (short nose, flat nasal bridge, wide lips, hypertelorism, ptosis, epicanthal folds, low-set ears, and low hairline) and limb anomalies (distal digital hypoplasia, absent nails, and altered palmar crease)

    (d) Fetal carbamazepine syndrome: resembles fetal hydantoin syndrome with addition of increased risk of spina bifida

    (e) Fetal phenobarbital syndrome is also similar to fetal hydantoin syndrome with addition of increased risk of hemorrhagic disease of newborn and neonatal withdrawal symptoms (irritability) after about 7 days of delivery

    (f) Fetal valproate syndrome: spina bifida, epicanthal folds, shallow orbits, hypertelorism, low-set ears, flat nasal bridge, upturned nasal tip, microcephaly, thin vermillion borders, downturned mouth, thin overlapping fingers and toes, and hyperconvex fingernails

4. Antidepressants

    (a) Tricyclic antidepressants (e.g. amitriptyline, imipramine) are associated with congenital malformations

        (i) Replaced by selective serotonin reuptake inhibitors (SSRIs) for first-line therapy for depression during pregnancy

    (b) No major risk for malformations and abnormalities with SSRIs

        (i) Paroxetine may be associated with increased risk for right ventricular outflow tract obstruction. Avoid paroxetine if possible and fetal echocardiography in women who used paroxetine during early pregnancy

    (c) Lithium is controversial during pregnancy.

        (i) Discontinuation is associated with higher chance of relapse of the affective disorder in 1 year.

        (ii) Can cause hypotonia, lethargy, and poor feeding in newborns.

5. Isotretinoin – treatment of cystic acne

    (a) Highly teratogenic: CNS malformations, microtia or anotia, micrognathia, cleft palate, cardiac and great vessel defects, thymic abnormalities, and eye anomalies

6. Warfarin

    (a) Fetal warfarin syndrome: nasal hypoplasia, depressed nasal bridge (often with a deep groove between the alae and nasal tip), stippled epiphyses, nail hypoplasia, mental retardation and growth restriction

    (b) Second and third trimester exposure can cause microcephaly, blindness, deafness, and growth restriction

7. Hyperthyroid medications

    (a) Propylthiouracil – can cause fetal and neonatal hypothyroidism and, rarely, goiter

    (b) Methimazole – Causes aplasia cutis congenital of the scalp in newborns

8. ACE inhibitors may increase cardiac and CNS defects. Can cause fetal renal failure and oligohydramnios, which may result in fetal limb contractures, craniofacial deformities, and pulmonary hypoplasia

9. Cyclophosphamide (chemotherapy) is associated with skeletal and palatal defects and with malformations of the limbs and eyes

10. Trimethoprim (antibiotic) antagonizes folic acid and increases risk of neural tube defects, cardiovascular defects, oral clefts, and urinary tract defects
11. Tetracyclines (antibiotic) bind to developing enamel and causes tooth discoloration
12. Aminoglycosides (antibiotic) are ototoxic for fetus
13. Corticosteroids
    (a) Commonly used for postoperative and chemotherapy-induced nausea and vomiting.
    (b) Associated with cleft lip with or without cleft palate when used before 10 weeks' gestation

Drug Effects on Newborn

17

1. In general, newborns are more sensitive than adults to the depressant effects of drugs
2. The seizure threshold is similar in newborns and adults
3. Newborns have larger volumes of distribution, requiring a higher dose of local anesthetic for toxic effects compared to adults
4. Changes in fetal heart rate after administration of local anesthetics are most often due to indirect effects (e.g. maternal hypotension and uterine hyperstimulation)
5. Preterm infant is more vulnerable than term infant to effects of analgesic and anesthetic drugs due to:
   (a) Less protein available for drug binding
   (b) Higher levels of bilirubin present and competing with drugs for protein binding
   (c) Greater access of drugs to the CNS due to poorly developed blood-brain barrier
   (d) Preterm infant has greater total body water and less fat content
   (e) Preterm infant has diminished ability to metabolize and excrete drugs
6. Neuraxial opioids have a favorable effect on neonatal outcome compared to systemic opioid
   (a) Better Apgar scores, and umbilical cord blood gas and pH measurements at delivery with neuraxial opioids compared to systemic opioids
   (b) Maternal epidural opioid administration by continuous infusion rarely results in drug accumulation and subsequent neonatal depression
   (c) Possible direct effect on the neonate at delivery due to systemic absorption and indirect effects by opioid-related maternal side effects (i.e., respiratory depression and hypoxemia)

© Springer Nature Switzerland AG 2019
C. Wasson et al., *Absolute Obstetric Anesthesia Review*,
https://doi.org/10.1007/978-3-319-96980-0_17

Amniotic Fluid

18

1. Amniocentesis – sampling of amniotic fluid
   (a) Most common indication during second trimester is cytogenetic analysis of fetal cells
      (i) Occasionally used to determine AFP levels and acetylcholinesterase activity to diagnose fetal neural tube defects
   (b) Not recommended prior to 15 weeks' gestation due to a high incidence of procedure-related pregnancy loss
   (c) Performed later in pregnancy for non-genetic indications:
      (i) Measures lecithin and sphingomyelin to assess fetal lung maturity
      (ii) Amnioreduction in pregnancies with severe polyhydramnios
      (iii) Confirm preterm rupture of membranes (PROM)
      (iv) Confirm or exclude an intra-amniotic infection
      (v) For spectrophotometric analysis of amniotic fluid bilirubin to determine fetal Rh type in pregnancies complicated by isoimmunization
2. Oligohydramnios – decreased amniotic fluid volume
   (a) In the latter half of pregnancy (and in the absence of ruptured membranes) reflects chronic uteroplacental insufficiency and/or increased renal artery resistance causing diminished urine output
   (b) Predisposes fetus to umbilical cord compression, which may cause intermittent fetal hypoxemia, meconium passage, or meconium aspiration
3. Polyhydramnios – increased amniotic fluid volume
   (a) Typically indicates fetal anatomic abnormalities (e.g., esophageal atresia)

© Springer Nature Switzerland AG 2019
C. Wasson et al., *Absolute Obstetric Anesthesia Review*,
https://doi.org/10.1007/978-3-319-96980-0_18

Antepartum Fetal Assessment and Therapy

19

1. Preterm (delivery <37 weeks) and posterm (delivery >42 weeks) are associated with higher perinatal and neonatal morbidity and mortality
2. Determination of gestational age
   (a) Most accurate in women undergoing in vitro fertilization
   (b) In women with regular menstrual cycles, Naegele's rule (subtract 3 months and add 7 days to last menstrual period) can be used
   (c) Uterine size (inaccurate in multiple gestations, uterine fibroids, or high BMI)
   (d) Fundal height in a singleton pregnancy should be at the umbilicus (approximately 20 cm above pubic symphysis) at 20 weeks.
   (e) Perception of fetal movement/quickening (occurs at 18–20 weeks in nulliparous women and 16–18 weeks in parous women)
   (f) Ultrasonography (crown-rump length in first trimester or fetal biometry during the second trimester)
3. Ultrasonography
   (a) Early ultrasound (US) improves accuracy of age dating
   (b) Detects pregnancy abnormalities (e.g., molar pregnancy), major fetal structural abnormalities (e.g., anencephaly), and multiple pregnancy
   (c) Allows estimation of birth weight
   (d) 3 types of examinations:
       (i) Basic – determines fetal number, viability, position, gestational age, and gross malformations
       (ii) Targeted/comprehensive – best performed at 18–20 weeks' gestation; fetal structures are examined to identify malformations
       (iii) Limited – used to answer specific questions (e.g., fetal viability, amniotic fluid volume, fetal presentation, placental location, cervical length) or to provide US guidance for procedures (e.g., amniocentesis)

© Springer Nature Switzerland AG 2019
C. Wasson et al., *Absolute Obstetric Anesthesia Review*,
https://doi.org/10.1007/978-3-319-96980-0_19

4. Fetal heart rate (FHR) monitoring
   (a) Should be performed at every visit
      (i) Low FHR (<100 bpm) is associated with increased risk of pregnancy loss, but may be due to congenital complete heart block, beta-adrenergic antagonists, hypoglycemia, hypothermia, or antithyroid medications
      (ii) Persistent fetal tachycardia (>160 bpm) is associated with fetal hypoxia, maternal fever, chorioamnionitis, administration of an anticholinergic or beta-adrenergic receptor agonist, fetal anemia, or tachyarrhythmia
5. Non-stress test (NST) a.k.a. fetal cardiotocography
   (a) Looks at FHR pattern with time and reflects the maturity of the fetal autonomic nervous system
      (i) Useful for cases of suspected uteroplacental insufficiency
      (ii) Less useful in extremely premature fetuses (<28 weeks) because the autonomic nervous system has not fully matured to influence the FHR
   (b) FHR and presence or absence of uterine contractions is recorded for 20–40 min. Evaluates:
      (i) Baseline FHR (normal is 110–160 bpm) and variability
      (ii) Presence of accelerations and periodic or episodic decelerations (early, variable, or late)
      (iii) Changes of FHR over time
   (c) NST is reported as reactive or nonreactive
      (i) Criteria for reactive NST:
         1. If <32 weeks, there should be 2 or more accelerations of at least 10 bpm for 10 s in a 20-min period
         2. If >32 weeks, there should be 2 or more accelerations of at least 15 bpm for 15 s in a 20-min period
      (ii) If above criteria are unmet, it is a nonreactive NST
   (d) Reactive NST: evidence of fetal health
   (e) Nonreactive NST: interpretation remains controversial (high false-positive rate)
6. Contraction Stress test (CST) a.k.a. oxytocin challenge test (OCT)
   (a) Assesses response of FHR to uterine contractions, usually induced by IV oxytocin or nipple stimulation
   (b) Requires a minimum of three minimal-moderate strength contractions in 10 min
   (c) Indirect evaluation of fetal oxygenation during periods of uterine contractions and diminished uteroplacental perfusion
      1. Better assessment of fetal well-being than either the NST or BPP
   (d) Negative CST (no decels with contractions) is reassuring
   (e) Positive CST (repetitive late or severe variable decels with contractions) suggests fetal hypoxia and is associated with adverse perinatal outcomes
   (f) Contraindications to CST: placenta previa, placental abruption, prior classic cesarean, and risk of preterm delivery

Table 19.1 Biophysical profile points

Variable	Normal (2 points)	Abnormal (0 points)
Fetal breathing movements	≥1 episode lasting ≥30 s	Absence or episode lasting <30 s
Gross body movements	≥3 discrete body/limb movements in 30 min	<3 episodes in 30 min
Fetal tone	≥1 active extension with return to flexion of fetal limbs or trunk	Slow extension with return to partial flexion, movement of limb in full extension, or absence of movement
Qualitative amniotic fluid volume	At least one pocket of amniotic fluid ≥1 cm	No amniotic fluid pockets or pocket <1 cm
Reactive nonstress test	≥ 2 FHR accelerations (≥15 bpm lasting ≥15 s in 30 min)	<2 episodes of FHR accelerations or accelerations <15 bpm over 30 min

7. Biophysical profile
   (a) Sonographic scoring system performed over a 30–40 min period to assess fetal well-being
   (b) 5 variables with 2 points each (2 if present, 0 if absent):
   (c) Score of 8–10 is reassuring; 4–6 requires further evaluation; 0–2 is non-reassuring and requires intervention/immediate delivery

8. Fetal therapy – Treatment may improve or correct in utero problems
   (a) Noninvasive
       (i) Antenatal corticosteroids for risk of imminent preterm birth between 23 and 24 to 34 weeks' gestation
       (ii) Strict glycemic control for pre-gestational diabetes mellitus
       (iii) Low-phenylalanine diet for phenylketonuria (autosomal recessive disorder due to phenylalanine hydroxylase deficiency)
       (iv) Maternal intravenous immunoglobulin ± corticosteroids for alloimmune thrombocytopenia
       (v) Maternal propylthiouracil for fetal thyrotoxicosis
       (vi) Maternal dexamethasone for congenital adrenal hyperplasia (usually due to 21-hydroxylase deficiency)
       (vii) Maternal digoxin for fetal supraventricular tachycardia
   (b) Invasive
       (i) Intrauterine transfusion for severe fetal anemia
       (ii) Fetal surgery for severe valvular stenosis, lung masses, congenital hydrocephalus, etc.
       (iii) Ex utero intrapartum therapy to allow intubation or other modes of oxygenation during delivery prior to ligation of the umbilical cord or to facilitate transition to ECMO

Systemic Medications: Opioids, Sedatives, Inhalational Agents

1. Opioids
   (a) Provide incomplete analgesia and have side effects (e.g. nausea, vomiting, delayed gastric emptying, dysphoria, drowsiness)
   (b) All opioids have low molecular weight and easily cross the placenta by diffusion
   (c) Opioids decrease fetal heart rate variability without worsening acid-base status
   (d) Metabolism and elimination of drugs are slower in neonates than adults
   (e) The blood-brain barrier is less well developed in the fetus and neonate than adults
   (f) Patient-controlled opioid analgesia (PCA)
      (i) Advantages of PCA (compared to IV boluses):
         1. Superior pain relief with lower doses of drug
         2. Less risk of maternal respiratory depression
         3. Less placental transfer of drug
         4. Less need for antiemetic agents
         5. Higher patient satisfaction

2. Sedatives
   (a) Barbiturates – sedative without any analgesic effect
      (i) Lipid soluble and readily cross placenta
   (b) Phenothiazines (e.g. promethazine or propiomazine) – provide sedation and decrease nausea and vomiting
      (i) Cross placenta and reduces FHR variability
      (ii) No evidence of neonatal respiratory depression
   (c) Benzodiazepines
      (i) Diazepam rapidly crosses the placenta and accumulates in the fetus. Diazepam has been associated with neonatal hypotonicity and respiratory depression and impairs neonatal thermoregulation

© Springer Nature Switzerland AG 2019
C. Wasson et al., *Absolute Obstetric Anesthesia Review*,
https://doi.org/10.1007/978-3-319-96980-0_20

Table 20.1 Systemic opioids used for labor analgesia

Drug	Usual dose	Onset	Duration (hours)	Comments
Meperidine	25–50 mg IV	5–10 min IV	2–3	Active metabolite with a long half life
	50–100 mg IM	40–45 min IM		Maximal neonatal depression 3–5 h after dose
Morphine	2–5 mg IV	10 min IV	3–4	More neonatal respiratory depression than meperidine
	5–10 mg IM	20–40 min IM		
				Active metabolite
Fentanyl	25–50 μg IV	2–3 min IV	30–60 min	Less neonatal depression than meperidine
Nalbuphine	10–20 mg IV or IM	2–3 min IV	3–6	Opioid agonist/antagonist
		15 min IM/SQ		Ceiling effect on respiratory depression
Butorphanol	1–2 mg IV or IM	5–10 min IV	4–6	Opioid agonist/antagonist
		30–60 min IM		Ceiling effect on respiratory depression
Tramadol	50–100 mg IV or IM	10 min IM	2–4	Less efficacious than meperidine
				More side effects than meperidine

Table 20.2 Most common PCA agents: meperidine, nalbuphine, fentanyl, and remifentanil

Drug	Patient-controlled dose	Lockout interval (min)
Meperidine	10–15 mg	8–20
Nalbuphine	1–3 mg	6–10
Fentanyl	10–25 μg	5–12
Remifentanil (bolus only)	0.2–0.8 μg/kg	2–3
Remifentanil (infusion with bolus dose)	Infusion: 0.025–0.1 μg/kg/min	2–3
	Bolus: 0.25 μg/kg	

3. Inhalational agents
    (a) Nitrous Oxide
        (i) Provides analgesia for labor, but does not completely eliminate the pain
        (ii) Does not interfere with uterine activity
        (iii) Does not depress neonatal respiration or neurobehavior
    (b) Volatile halogenated agents
        (i) All agents cause a dose-related relaxation of uterine smooth muscle
        (ii) Concentrations >0.5 MAC are not recommended when uterine tone is desired (e.g., after delivery)

Epidural, Caudal, Spinal, Combined Spinal/Epidural

21

1. Pain during first stage of labor due to distention of lower uterine segment and cervix (nerve fibers T10-L1)
2. Pain during second stage of labor due to distention of the vagina and perineum (pudendal nerve and S2-4)
   (a) These nerve fibers are larger and may require administration of a more concentrated solution and/or a greater volume of local anesthetic for adequate blockade (e.g. 5–10 ml of 1–2% lidocaine or 0.25% bupivacaine)
   (b) The sitting position helps facilitate the onset of perineal analgesia
3. Effective epidural analgesia:
   (a) Reduces maternal catecholamines, which can improve uteroplacental perfusion and cause more effective uterine activity
   (b) Blunts maternal hyperventilation from painful uterine contractions, which then decreases maternal respiratory alkalosis, leading to a rightward shift of the oxyhemoglobin dissociation curve, causing decreased maternal Hgb affinity for O_2 and increased O_2 delivery to the fetus
4. A specific cervical dilation is not required prior to placing an epidural for labor analgesia. All that is needed is active labor and patient request.
   (a) Late first stage of labor (i.e. >8 cm dilation) is also not a contraindication for epidural placement, especially in a nulliparous woman.
   (b) Consider opioid-only spinal anesthesia for multiparous women in late stages of labor as it is quicker onset and will cover the sacral nerves.
5. Contraindications for neuraxial techniques:
   (a) Patient refusal or inability to cooperate
   (b) Increased intracranial pressure as a result of a mass lesion, which may predispose the patient to brainstem herniation after dural puncture
   (c) Skin or soft tissue infection at the site of needle puncture
   (d) Frank coagulopathy
   (e) Uncorrected maternal hypovolemia
   (f) Inadequate training or inexperience in the technique

© Springer Nature Switzerland AG 2019
C. Wasson et al., *Absolute Obstetric Anesthesia Review*,
https://doi.org/10.1007/978-3-319-96980-0_21

6. Steps to prepare for neuraxial labor analgesia:
   (a) Review of parturient's OB history
   (b) Focused pre-anesthetic evaluation that includes maternal OB, anesthetic, and health history
   (c) Brief physical exam (i.e. vital signs, airway, heart, lungs, and back)
   (d) Ideally FHR should be monitored before, during, and after neuraxial placement if possible. However, if not possible, then it should be monitored before and after the initiation of neuraxial analgesia.
   (e) Resuscitation equipment (O_2 source, suction source, AMBU bag, face masks, oral airways, laryngoscope and blades, ETT, bougie), drugs (sedative-hypnotic agents (thiopental, propofol, ketamine, midazolam), succinylcholine, ephedrine, epinephrine, phenylephrine, atropine, calcium chloride, sodium bicarbonate, naloxone), and supplies must be immediately available for the management of serious complications of epidural analgesia (e.g. hypotension, total spinal anesthesia, systemic local anesthetic toxicity)

7. After initiation of neuraxial analgesia, patient's oxygen saturation should be monitored continuously and blood pressure assessed every 3–5 min for the first 30 min or until mother is hemodynamically stable, then every 15 min for another 60 min, then a minimum of once every 60 min thereafter while epidural infusion is in use.

8. Routine measurement of platelet count is not necessary, but should be individualized and based on a patient's history (e.g., preeclampsia with severe features), physical examination, and clinical signs.

9. Correction of hypovolemia with IV fluids is necessary before the initiation of neuraxial analgesia to prevent hypotension from sympathetic blockade
   (a) Most anesthesia providers administer approximately 500 mL of lactated ringers
   (b) The ASA states that a fixed volume of fluids is not required before neuraxial analgesia is initiated
   (c) Preloading or co-loading IV fluids can decrease the incidence of hypotension, but it is not routine practice and should be guided by assessment of intravascular fluid status.
   (d) Fluid should be administered cautiously in patients at risk for pulmonary edema (e.g., renal disease, heart disease, severe preeclampsia)

10. Patient position: sitting vs lateral decubitus
    (a) Lateral advantages:
        (i) Less risk of orthostatic hypotension
        (ii) Position facilitates continuous FHR monitoring during placement of epidural catheter
        (iii) Some patients find it more comfortable
    (b) Sitting position is advantageous in obese women due to:
        (i) Better respiratory mechanics
        (ii) Facilitation of identification of midline and bony landmarks
        (iii) Maternal comfort during placement of epidural catheter

11. Initiation of epidural analgesia
    (a) Place epidural catheter in epidural space
    (b) Administer test dose to rule out intrathecal or IV placement of catheter
        (i) Negative response does not guarantee correct placement of the epidural catheter in the epidural space, nor does it guarantee the catheter is not malpositioned in a blood vessel or subarachnoid space (e.g. patients on beta-blockers will not have a tachycardic response)
        (ii) Increase in HR of 20 bpm within 45 s of test dose containing 15 ug of epinephrine (3 ml of 1:200,000 solution) is 100% sensitive and specific for IV injection. Increase in SBP of 15–25 mmHg may also be observed.
        (iii) Aspiration of a multiorifice epidural catheter for blood has a 98% sensitivity for detection of intravascular location
        (iv) Perform sensory, motor, and sympathetic function test 3–5 min after test dose before concluding that the intrathecal test dose is negative
    (c) If test dose is negative, secure epidural catheter
    (d) Administer 5–15 mL of epidural local anesthetic in 5 mL increments
    (e) Monitor maternal BP every 3–5 min and oxygen saturation and heart rate continuously for the first 30 min
    (f) Assess pain score and extent of sensory blockade (both cephalad and caudad)
    (g) Initiate maintenance epidural analgesia
12. Steps to minimize local anesthetic toxicity (LAST):
    (a) Observe for passive return of CSF or blood in catheter
    (b) Administer test dose between contractions
    (c) Aspirate before administering any dose
    (d) Administer doses incrementally
    (e) Maintain verbal contact with the patient
    (f) Assess for an appropriate level and density of sensory and motor blockade
13. Caudal anesthesia is used infrequently, but is a good choice for the second stage of labor in selected patients in whom lumbar epidural is hazardous or contraindicated (e.g., patients with prior spine surgery)
14. Choice of local anesthetic
    (a) Ideal analgesic drug for labor:
        (i) Rapid onset of effective analgesia with minimal motor blockade
        (ii) Minimal risk of maternal toxicity
        (iii) Negligible effect on uterine activity and uteroplacental perfusion
        (iv) Limited transplacental transfer (minimal direct effect on fetus)
        (v) Long duration of action
    (b) Intrathecal opioids effectively relieve the visceral pain of the early first stage of labor, but must be combined with a local anesthetic to relieve the somatic pain of the late first stage and the second stage of labor
    (c) Addition of opioid to local anesthetic shortens latency, prolongs the duration of analgesia, improves the quality of analgesia, reduces shivering, decreases the overall local anesthetic dose, and increases patient satisfaction

(i) Advantages of lower local anesthetic dose:
  1. Decreased risk of systemic LAST
  2. Decreased risk of high or total spinal
  3. Decreased plasma concentration of local anesthetic in the fetus and neonate
  4. Decreased intensity of motor blockade
(d) Spinal anesthesia
  (i) Lidocaine is short to intermediate duration
  (ii) Bupivacaine, tetracaine, levobupivacaine, and ropivacaine are intermediate to long
  (iii) Opioid is often added to improve the quality of anesthesia and provide post-op analgesia
    1. Also decreases the incidence of intra-op nausea and vomiting
    2. Combination of morphine, bupivacaine, and fentanyl shortens latency of onset, prolongs duration of analgesia, and decreases analgesic use in the first 24 h postpartum compared to bupivacaine and fentanyl without morphine.
  (iv) Administering opioid alone intrathecal provides complete analgesia without a sympathectomy or motor blockade (useful in patients who won't tolerate a decrease in preload (e.g. stenotic heart lesions)).
    1. Administering fentanyl >25 mcg causes increased side effects (i.e. pruritus, respiratory depression) without increased analgesia
(e) Epidural anesthesia
  (i) Longer-acting agents (e.g., bupivacaine, ropivacaine, levobupivacaine) are used for maintenance of epidural labor analgesia; shorter-acting agents (e.g., 2% lidocaine) are used for epidural surgical anesthesia
  (ii) Bupivacaine
    1. Most popular due to differential sensory blockade, long duration of action, low frequency of tachyphylaxis, and low cost
    2. Risk of cardiac toxicity/arrest after unintentional intravascular injection
  (iii) Ropivacaine
    1. Less cardiac toxicity and greater differential sensory blockade than bupivacaine
    2. Less motor block than bupivacaine
  (iv) Levobupivacaine
    1. Not available in US
    2. Better safety profile than bupivacaine
  (v) 2% lidocaine with epinephrine is used for epidural anesthesia for cesarean delivery
    1. Addition of epinephrine (5 ug/ml) causes a modest prolongation of the block and improves quality of epidural lidocaine anesthesia.
    2. May also add fentanyl (50–100 mcg) or sufentanil (5–10 mcg) for a denser block with better blockade of visceral stimulation

3. Not used for labor epidural due to shorter duration of action compared to bupivacaine, ropivacaine, and levobupivacaine

   (vi) 2-chloroprocaine

     1. Faster onset than lidocaine. When time is of the essence, this is the drug of choice. Even though it has the highest pKa (8.9), its onset of action is rapid because it is used in high concentration.

     2. Rapidly metabolized by plasma esterases, therefore less likely to have serious adverse consequences if there is an unintentional intravascular injection

     3. May interefere with subsequent administration of opioids and bupivacaine, although this possibility is controversial

(f) Caudal anesthesia

   (i) Useful for patients in whom access to the lumbar spinal canal is not possible (e.g. due to fused lumbar spine)

   (ii) Drugs identical to those used for lumbar epidural, however much larger volume (e.g. 25–30 ml) of local anesthetic is required for labor analgesia or cesarean delivery.

   (iii) Since the caudal epidural space is more vascular and larger volumes are required, the risk of LAST is increased

15. Equipment and Needle and Catheter Placement

  (a) Continuous spinal technique: Large-bore epidural needle and catheter are used, which increases risk of post-dural puncture headache

    (i) Option for patients with unintentional dural puncture

  (b) Single-shot spinal technique is preferred over continuous spinal anesthesia for most OB pts.

  (c) Cutting-bevel needles (Quincke) are rarely used in OB anesthesia due to increased incidence of post-dural puncture headache

  (d) Non-cutting needles (Whitacre, Sprotte, and Greene) are used instead for spinal anesthesia

  (e) Needle advancement should stop if the patient complains of pain during any nerve block technique

    (i) Pain or paresthesias may result from needle contact with central nerves or the spinal cord

    (ii) If paresthesias resolve, local anesthetic may be injected

    (iii) If paresthesias persist, withdraw and reposition the needle

    (iv) NEVER inject local anesthetic if the patient complains of paresthesias or sharp pain, as these may signal injection into a nerve or the spinal cord

  (f) An epidural catheter initially placed in the epidural space can migrate into a vein or the subdural or subarachnoid space

    (i) Inappropriately high level of anesthesia signals the administration of an excessive dose of local anesthetic or subdural or subarachnoid migration of the catheter

    (ii) A low level of anesthesia signals IV migration of the catheter, movement of the catheter outside the epidural space, or administration of inadequate dose of local anesthesia

(g) During epidural placement, the needle should be advanced into the inter-spinous ligament, or even into the ligamentum flavum, before the loss-of-resistance syringe is attached. This has three advantages:
  (i) Encourages use of proprioception while directing and advancing the needle
  (ii) Shortens time required for successful identification of epidural space
  (iii) Lowers likelihood of false-positive loss of resistance
(h) Combined spinal-epidural has advantages of both spinal and epidural anesthesia (quick onset and long duration)
(i) The sacrococcygeal ligament is an extension of the ligamentum flavum and overlies the sacral hiatus

16. Side effects of neuraxial anesthesia
  (a) Hypotension is due to sympathetic blockade, which causes peripheral vasodilation and increases venous capacitance
    (i) Uncorrected hypotension leads to decreased uteroplacental perfusion as perfusion depends on normal maternal blood pressure (BP)
    (ii) Severe and prolonged hypotension leads to hypoxia and acidosis in the fetus
    (iii) Prevention: avoidance of aortocaval compression and IV fluids
    (iv) Treatment: additional IV fluids and full lateral and Trendelenburg position of mother
      1. If hypotension persists after IV fluids and positioning, if it is severe, or if the FHR is non-reassuring, administer IV vasopressors (e.g. ephedrine 5–10 mg or phenylephrine 50–100 mcg)
      2. Phenylephrine has been shown to have higher umbilical artery blood pH at birth
  (b) Pruritus – the most common side effect of neuraxial opioids (higher incidence in spinals than epidurals)
    (i) Treatment: most effective is a centrally acting μ-opioid antagonist (e.g., naloxone or naltrexone) or a partial agonist-antagonist (e.g., nalbuphine), but may decrease the analgesia.
      1. Naloxone: 40–80 μg IV bolus or 1–2 μg/kg/h continuous IV infusion
      2. Nalbuphine: 2.5–5 mg IV bolus
      3. Naltrexone 6 mg PO
    (ii) Antihistamines (e.g., diphenhydramine) are usually ineffective because the pruritus is not due to histamine release. Any observed effect is likely due to the sedating effects.
    (iii) Prophylactic ondansetron may decrease opioid-induced pruritus, as may sub-hypnotic doses of propofol (10–20 mg)
  (c) Nausea and vomiting can be due to hypotension due to neuroblockade, pregnancy itself, pain, opioid-induced delay of gastric emptying, and systemic opioids
    (i) Treatment: metoclopramide, ondansetron, and droperidol

   (d) Fever – increase in core temp (>1 °C, with a T_{max} of 38 °C)
      (i) Mechanisms remains unclear
      (ii) Epidural analgesia may alter maternal thermoregulation by raising
           core temperature that is tolerated and preventing sweating and evapo-
           rative heat loss in levels with blockade
      (iii) Inflammatory response is noninfectious in etiology
   (e) Shivering is often associated with normothermia and vasodilation, suggest-
       ing a non-thermoregulatory cause
   (f) Urinary retention is due to blockade of sacral nerve roots
   (g) Recrudescence of HSV
   (h) Delayed gastric emptying

Paracervical Block, Lumbar Sympathetic Block, Pudendal Block

22

1. Paracervical block
   (a) Performed by OB, not anesthesia
   (b) Provides analgesia for first stage of labor
   (c) Does not affect progression of labor
   (d) Does not block somatic sensory fibers from lower vagina, vulva, and perineum, so it does not relieve pain during late first stage and second stage of labor
   (e) Maternal complications:
       (i) Vasovagal syncope
       (ii) Laceration of the vaginal mucosa
       (iii) LAST
       (iv) Parametrial hematoma
       (v) Postpartum neuropathy
       (vi) Paracervical, retropsoal, or subgluteal abscess
   (f) Fetal complications
       (i) Direct injection of local anesthetic into the fetal scalp can cause LAST and fetal death
       (ii) Bradycardia is the most common fetal complication. The etiology is unclear. There are four theories:
           1. Reflex bradycardia due to manipulation of the fetal head, the uterus, or the uterine blood vessels
           2. Direct fetal CNS and myocardial depression due to rapid absorption of local anesthetic into the uteroplacental circulation
           3. Increased uterine activity from systemic local anesthetic absorption leading to decreased uteroplacental perfusion
           4. Uterine and/or umbilical artery vasoconstriction due to direct vasoconstrictive effect of local anesthetic

© Springer Nature Switzerland AG 2019
C. Wasson et al., *Absolute Obstetric Anesthesia Review*,
https://doi.org/10.1007/978-3-319-96980-0_22

2. Lumbar sympathetic block
   (a) Provides analgesia during the first stage of labor, but not the second
   (b) Good option for patients with a history of previous back surgery that prevents successful epidural
   (c) Complications:
       (i) Maternal hypotension – reduced by giving 500 mL of Lactated ringers IV prior to the block
       (ii) Systemic local anesthetic toxicity if accidently injected into blood vessel
       (iii) Total spinal anesthesia if accidently injected into intrathecal space
       (iv) Retroperitoneal hematoma
       (v) Horner's syndrome
       (vi) Post-dural puncture headache
   (d) Fetal complications are rare
3. Pudendal block
   (a) Pudendal nerve made of anterior divisions of the 2nd, 3rd, and 4th sacral nerves and is the primary source of sensory innervation for the lower vagina, vulva, and perineum
   (b) Good for second stage of labor
   (c) Maternal complications are uncommon
       (i) Systemic local anesthetic toxicity from direct intravascular injection or systemic absorption of an excessive dose
       (ii) Vaginal, ischiorectal, and retroperitoneal hematomas from trauma to the pudendal artery
       (iii) Subgluteal and retropsoal abscesses
   (d) Fetal complications are rare

1. Unintentional dural puncture
   (a) Occurs in approximately 1.5% of OB patients
   (b) Approximately 52% will experience post-dural puncture headache with a 17 gauge touhy needle
      (i) Risk decreases with smaller needles
      (ii) Risk decreased with pencil point needles compared to cutting needles
   (c) To minimize incidence of unintentional dural puncture:
      (i) Identify the ligamentum flavum during epidural needle advancement
      (ii) Understand the likely depth of the epidural space in an individual patient (Table 23.1)
      (iii) Advance the needle between contractions, when unexpected patient movement is less likely
      (iv) Adequately control the needle-syringe assembly during advancement of the needle
      (v) Clear the needle of clotted blood or bone plugs
   (d) Management
      (i) Place the epidural catheter within the subarachnoid space and use as a continuous spinal anesthetic technique
         1. Increased risk of total spinal due to risk of mistaking spinal catheter for epidural catheter
      (ii) Or place new catheter in another lumbar interspace
         1. Local anesthetic or opioid injected through the epidural may pass through the dural puncture site and into the subarachnoid space
2. Unintentional intravascular or subarachnoid injection
   (a) Pregnant women are at higher risk for unintentional intravenous cannulation due to engorged epidural veins
   (b) Unintentional intravascular or subarachnoid injection can be life-threatening, so several precautions must be taken:

© Springer Nature Switzerland AG 2019
C. Wasson et al., *Absolute Obstetric Anesthesia Review*,
https://doi.org/10.1007/978-3-319-96980-0_23

Table 23.1 Typical distance to epidural space for each spinal level

	Distance (cm)		
	Median	5th %ile	95th %ile
L1–2	4.23	3.12	6.33
L2–3	4.86	3.29	7.32
L3–4	4.93	3.57	7.44
L4–5	4.78	3.25	6.75

    (i) Aspiration prior to every injection
    (ii) Incremental administration of small amounts of drug
    (iii) Use an infusion when appropriate
    (iv) Administration of epidural test dose
      1. The test dose contains epinephrine, which causes a transient increase in HR (15–20 bpm) within the first minute
      2. The test dose is less specific in laboring women due to cyclic changes in maternal heart rate
        (a) Distinguish tachycardia due to contractions versus IV epinephrine by giving the test dose right after a contraction
(c) Management of total spinal anesthesia:
    (i) Administer 100% O_2 to maintain maternal oxygenation
    (ii) Provide positive-pressure ventilation
    (iii) Avoid aortocaval compression
    (iv) Monitor maternal vitals, EKG, and FHR
    (v) Support maternal BP with fluids and vasopressors
(d) Management of unintentional IV injection of local anesthetic:
    (i) Same as that for total spinal with the following additions
    (ii) Prevent maternal respiratory and metabolic acidosis
    (iii) Initiate ACLS if necessary
    (iv) Treat seizures with a barbiturate or a benzodiazepine as hypoxemia and acidosis can quickly develop
    (v) Avoid propofol in patients having signs of cardiovascular instability
    (vi) Management of arrhythmias:
      1. Do not treat with lidocaine as LA toxicity is additive
      2. Amrinone is superior to epinephrine in improving contractility depression by bupivacaine (keep epinephrine <1 ug/kg)
      3. Avoid vasopressin, Ca++ blocking agents, beta blockers
    (vii) Consider administering 20% lipid emulsion (1.5 mL/kg bolus followed by 0.25–0.5 mL/kg/min infusion). Continue infusion for at least 10 min after attaining circulatory stability.
    (viii) Prepare for emergency delivery, including cesarean delivery, if mother is not resuscitated within 4 min (delivery may facilitate successful resuscitation of the mother)

3. Inadequate anesthesia (inadequate extent of sensory block, non-uniform block, or inadequate density of block)
   (a) When evaluating breakthrough pain, evaluate extent of bilateral sensory blockade in both cephalad and caudad directions
      (i) If extent of block is inadequate, bolus the epidural with 5–15 mL of dilute local anesthetic and increase the rate of the maintenance infusion
      (ii) If block is asymmetric, bolus the epidural with 5–15 mL of dilute local anesthetic and increase the rate of the maintenance infusion, place the less blocked side in dependent position.
      (iii) If boluses do not provide adequate pain relief, replace the epidural
   (b) No blockade requires replacement of epidural catheter
   (c) Pain becomes more intense as labor progresses. A bolus of local anesthetic may be needed as the patient progresses.
      (i) May require increasing the concentration of the maintenance local anesthetic infusion
   (d) Rule out other causes of pain (e.g., distended bladder or ruptured uterus)
4. Respiratory depression is due to opioid administration
   (a) Lipid-soluble opioids (e.g. fentanyl or sufentanil) have a short "time window" for respiratory depression (within 2 h).
   (b) Hydrophilic opioids (e.g. morphine) has a delayed onset and may not occur until 6–12 h post injection of drug
5. Extensive motor blockade may occur after repeated boluses or after many hours of a continuous infusion of local anesthetic
   (a) May impair maternal expulsive efforts during the second stage of labor and increase the likelihood of instrumental delivery
   (b) Discontinue the infusion for a short period (e.g. 30 min) and then restart at a reduced rate or with a more dilute solution of local anesthetic
6. Prolonged neuroblockade is typically due to high concentration of local anesthetic
7. Epidural hematoma
   (a) Factors that argue against an epidural hematoma:
      (i) Absence of back pain
      (ii) Unilateral block
      (iii) Regression (rather than progression) of the symptoms
8. Back pain occurs in approximately 50% of women during pregnancy and the puerperium
   (a) Risk factors include antepartum back pain and inability to reduce weight to prepregnancy levels
   (b) There is no significant relationship between epidural analgesia and long-term backache
   (c) There is no difference in incidence of postpartum backache between women who delivered with or without an epidural

9. Aspiration
   (a) Maternal mortality has recently declined due to greater use of neuraxial anesthesia; use of antacids, histamine (H2) antagonists, and/or PPIs; use of RSI for GA; improvement in training of anesthesia providers; and enforcement of NPO policies
   (b) Morbidity and mortality vary according to:
      (i) Physical status of the patient
      (ii) The type of aspirate (particulate matter is more severe)
      (iii) The volume of aspirate (larger volumes have higher mortality)
      (iv) The therapy administered
      (v) The criteria for making the diagnosis
   (c) Risk factors for aspiration pneumonitis: aspirate pH<2.5 and volume >25 mL
   (d) Acidic liquid injures the alveolar epithelium, leading to alveolar exudate composed of edema, albumin, fibrin, cellular debris, and RBCs
      (i) Exudative pulmonary edema, bronchial obstruction from cellular debris, reduced lung compliance, and shunting result in hypoxemia, increased pulmonary vascular resistance, and increased work of breathing
      (ii) Patient may develop acute lung injury (ALI) or adult respiratory distress syndrome (ARDS)
         1. Clinical signs: acute onset of respiratory distress
         2. Biochemical signs: PaO2/FiO2 ratio less than 300 for ALI or less than 200 for ARDS
         3. Radiographic signs: bilateral diffuse fluffy alveolar infiltrates
   (e) Management:
      (i) Rigid bronchoscopy and lavage
         1. Suction upper airway, intubate, suction primary bronchi
         2. Rigid bronchoscopy is useful to remove large food particles
         3. Lavage with saline or bicarbonate does not reduce damage and may worsen preexisting hypoxemia
      (ii) Antibiotics should only be considered if signs of infection are present (e.g., fever, worsening infiltrates on CXR, leukocytosis, positive Gram stain of sputum, clinical deterioration)
         1. Prophylactic use may lead to development of resistant organisms
      (iii) Management of hypoxemia with CPAP in non-intubated patients and PEEP in intubated patients
      (iv) Corticosteroids do not have supportive evidence for use
   (f) Prophylaxis: nonparticulate antacids, H2-antagonsits, and/or metoclopramide
   (g) Sellick Maneuver (AKA cricoid pressure) – maintain until the endotracheal tube's cuff is inflated and position is confirmed.
      (i) Assumes the esophagus lies directly posterior to the cricoid cartilage and can be effectively occluded
      (ii) Esophagus is often displaced laterally with cricoid pressure
   (h) The most effective way to decrease the risk of aspiration is to avoid the administration of general anesthesia

10. Postpartum headache has multiple causes. Differential diagnosis:
   (a) Primary headaches:
      (i) Migraine – pulsating pain in a unilateral location, nausea, photophobia
      (ii) Tension-type headache – bilateral, nonpulsating, and **NOT** aggravated by physical activity
      (iii) Cluster headache
      (iv) Trigeminal autonomic cephalgias
   (b) Secondary headaches
      (i) Musculoskeletal – accompanied by neck and shoulder pain
      (ii) Preeclampsia/eclampsia– often bilateral, pulsating, and aggravated by physical activity
      (iii) Post-dural puncture headache (PDPH) – occurs within 5 days of dural puncture and lasts less than 1 week
         1. Pain in frontal and occipital regions
         2. Neck stiffness
         3. Postural component (worse with standing, improved with lying flat)
         4. Other symptoms: tinnitus, hypacusis, photophobia, nausea
         5. Occasionally cranial nerve palsy occurs (most frequently CN VI), leading to the inability to abduct the eye and diplopia
         6. Risk factors:
            (a) Age – uncommon in patients >60; most common in age 20–40
            (b) Gender – women 2× as likely as men
            (c) Vaginal delivery – likely due to expulsive efforts during second stage of labor
            (d) Morbid obesity is protective
            (e) Airplane travel
            (f) History of previous post-dural headache
            (g) Multiple dural punctures
            (h) Neuraxial anesthetic technique:
               (i) Cutting needle has increased risk compared to pencil-point, non-cutting needle
               (ii) Larger needle has increased risk
         7. Prevention of post-dural puncture headache after unintentional dural puncture:
            (a) No benefit of bed rest over early immobilization
            (b) No benefit of increased hydration
            (c) Tight abdominal binder placed after delivery and continued until discharge home reduces incidence of PDPH
            (d) Caffeine has no benefit
            (e) Prophylactic neuraxial opioids do not reduce PDPH
            (f) Intrathecal catheter placement after unintentional dural puncture reduce incidence of PDPH if left in place for 24 h post-delivery

8. Treatment of PDPH
    (a) Conservative management for the first 24 h:
        (i) Bed rest
        (ii) Oral analgesics
        (iii) Psychological support
    (b) Pharmacologic treatment – caffeine, sumatriptan, ACTH (for refractory PDPHs), oral gabapentin
    (c) PDPH refractory to conservative measures: epidural blood patch – 12–20 mL autologous blood injected into the epidural space. "Gold standard" therapy. As many as 29% of patients may require a second epidural blood patch
        (iv) Spontaneous intracranial hypotension – same signs/symptoms of post-dural puncture headache without a history of dural trauma
        (v) Pneumocephalus – frontal headache with abrupt onset **IMMEDIATELY** following dural puncture; symptoms worsen with standing
        (vi) Cortical vein thrombosis – nonspecific headache +/− postural component; often accompanied by focal neurological signs and seizures
        (vii) Subarachnoid hemorrhage – abrupt onset of intense and incapacitating headache; often unilateral; accompanied by nausea, nuchal rigidity, and altered consciousness
        (viii) Subdural hematoma – accompanied by focal neurologic signs and/or altered consciousness
        (ix) Cerebral infarction/ischemia – moderate headache with focal neurological signs and/or altered consciousness
        (x) Posterior reversible (leuko)encephalopathy syndrome (PRES) – severe and diffuse headache with acute or gradual onset; possible focal neurologic deficits and seizures
        (xi) Brain tumor – progressive headache; worse in the morning; aggravated by coughing/straining
        (xii) Pseudotumor cerebri/benign intracranial HTN – progressive nonpulsating headache; aggravated by coughing/straining
        (xiii) Sinusitis – frontal headache with accompanying pain in the face; accompanied by nasal discharge, anosmia, and fever
        (xiv) Meningitis – diffuse headache associated with nausea, photophobia, phonophobia, general malaise, and fever
        (xv) Caffeine withdrawal – bilateral and pulsating; occur within 24 h of cessation of regular caffeine consumption
        (xvi) Lactation headache – associated with onset of breast-feeding or with breast engorgement
11. Neurologic complications of pregnancy and neuraxial anesthesia
    (a) Complications from neuraxial anesthesia may be immediate or they may be prolonged or delayed
    (b) Obstetric sources are the most common cause of postpartum nerve injury due to compression of nerves in the pelvis by the fetal head or from more distal compression

(c) Abnormal presentation, persistent occiput posterior position, fetal macrosomia, breakthrough pain during epidural labor analgesia, a prolonged second stage of labor, difficult instrumental delivery, and prolonged use of the lithotomy position may be risk factors for postpartum neuropathy

(d) Compression of the lumbosacral trunk (L4-L5) by the fetal head at the pelvic brim is probably the most common cause of postpartum footdrop and L5 dermatome sensory disturbances, typically seen after prolonged labor and difficult vaginal delivery

(e) The obturator nerve (L2-L4) is also vulnerable to compressive injury as it crosses the brim of the pelvis. Pain may happen when damage occurs, followed by weakness of hip adduction and internal rotation and sensory disturbance over the upper inner thigh.

(f) Femoral nerve (L2–L4) does not enter the pelvis, therefore is not vulnerable to compression by the fetal head, but is susceptible to stretch injury as it passes beneath the inguinal ligament. Femoral nerve palsy may result from prolonged flexion, abduction, and external rotation of the hips during the second stage of labor.
   (i) Ability to walk on a level surface is preserved, but possible loss of ability to climb stairs
   (ii) Diminished or absent patellar reflex

(g) Meralgia paresthetica is neuropathy of the lateral femoral cutaneous nerve (purely sensory nerve)– numbness, tingling or burning of the anteriolateral aspect of the thigh
   (i) Associated with increased intra-abdominal pressure typically starting at about 30 weeks' gestation or by retractors used during pelvic surgery.

(h) Sciatic nerve palsy may arise from compression of the nerve, usually in the buttock
   (i) Occurs during childbirth typically from sitting in one position too long or from a hip wedge misplaced during cesarean delivery. Hypotension may be contributory.
   (ii) Causes loss of sensation and movement distal to the knee with sparing of the medial side.

(i) The common peroneal nerve is vulnerable to compression as it passes around the fibular head distal to the knee.
   (i) Due to:
      1. Prolonged squatting in "natural childbirth"
      2. Excessive knee flexion
      3. Compression of the lateral side of the knee by parturient's or partner's hand, or
      4. Prolonged lithotomy position.
   (ii) Manifests as sensory impairment on the anterolateral calf and dorsum of the foot
      1. Foot drop may occur and be profound
      2. Plantar flexion and inversion at the ankle are preserved

   (j) Postpartum bladder dysfunction

     (i) Significant factors for postpartum bladder dysfunction: prolonged second stage of labor, instrumental delivery, and perineal damage

    (ii) Multiple causes of urinary retention or incontinence:

       1. Cauda equina syndrome due to trauma to the conus, a space-occupying lesion, or subarachnoid neurotoxicity

       2. Traumatic delivery causing damage to the pelvic floor, intrapelvic nerve damage, and/or urethral swelling or damage

   (iii) There is a weak correlation between epidural analgesia and increased residual volume in the postpartum period

  (k) CNS lesions may be due to neuraxial block, or may have other causes, such as a prolapsed intervertebral disc

     (i) Headaches (see above)

    (ii) Cranial nerve palsy – May arise from major loss of CSF after unintentional dural puncture with a large needle.

       1. Most often abducent nerve (CN VI) because of its long course within the cranium making it the most vulverable CN

       2. Facial nerve (CN VII) and CN VIII palsy may also occur. Tinnitus from CN VIII dysfunction may become permanent

       3. All cranial nerve palsies require a prompt epidural blood patch

   (iii) Cranial subdural hematoma from ruptured bridging meningeal veins due to reduced CSF pressure

       1. Suspect when headache persists after dural puncture and treatment with an epidural blood patch (especially if accompanied by altered consciousness, seizures, or other focal neurological finds)

       2. Diagnose with MRI

       3. May be fatal without urgent diagnosis and surgery

   (iv) Anterior spinal artery syndrome may occur when an epidural catheter migrates into the same foramen occupied by the artery of Adamkiewcz (typically originates on the left side of the aorta between T8–L1)

       1. The condition resolves rapidly and completely if the catheter is withdrawn before permanent damage has occurred

    (v) Damage to conus medullaris may occur with spinal anesthesia. Patient typically complains of pain on needle insertion prior to injection of fluid, often followed by normal appearance of (CSF) from needle hub, easy injection of local anesthetic, and normal onset of neural blockade

   (vi) Space-occupying lesions (i.e., intraspinal hematomas (epidural or subdural), epidural abscess, and intraspinal tumors) can cause dangerous compression of nervous tissue and its blood supply

       1. Urgent laminectomy (within 6–12 h of symptom onset) is required to avoid permanent neurologic damage

       2. Signs and symptoms depend on vertebral level

         (a) Lower thoracic lesions: leg weakness or paraplegia

         (b) Lumbar lesions: cauda equine syndrome, including urinary retention and incontinence

Table 23.2 Comparison of epidural abscess and meningitis

	Entry point	Usual causative agent	Possible source of infection	Risk factors
Epidural abscess	Through the catheter or along its tissue track	*Staphylococcus aureus*	Patient's skin; epidural equipment contaminated by operator's skin; body fluids in the bed	Prolonged catheterization; poor aseptic technique; multiple insertion attempts; traumatic insertion; lying in a wet, contaminated bed; immunocompromised (steroids, diabetes, AIDS)
Meningitis	Blood, via the dural puncture	*Streptococcus viridans*	Vagina; blood-borne; talking without a mask; anesthesia provider's oral cavity	Dural puncture; labor; anesthesia provider not wearing a mask; vaginal infection; bacteremia

      3. Risk factors for epidural hematoma: difficult or traumatic epidural needle/catheter placement; coagulopathy or therapeutic anticoagulation; spinal deformity; and spinal tumor (Table 23.2)

(vii) Comparison of epidural abscess and meningitis

    1. Epidural abscess

      (a) Symptoms typically begin 4–10 days after removal of the catheter

      (b) Severe backache (with local tenderness) and fever, with or without radiating or root pain

      (c) Untreated, symptoms progress to leg weakness, paresthesias, bladder dysfunction, or other evidence of cauda equine syndrome

      (d) *Staphylococcus aureus* is the most common cause of epidural abscess, which enters via the skin. Therefore, sterile gloves, aseptic prep, and proper drape technique are imperative.

      (e) Treatment: prompt laminectomy and antibiotic therapy for 2–4 weeks.

      (f) Diagnostic lumbar puncture is contraindicated

    2. Meningitis

      (a) Community-acquired is caused by *N. meningitides, S. pneumoniae, or H. influenza,* but post-spinal meningitis is caused by *S. viridans* (normal flora of upper airway and vagina. This is why it is important to wear a mask)

      (b) Presentation: fever, headache, photophobia, nausea, vomiting, and neck stiffness

      (c) Diagnosis by lumbar puncture (increased CSF pressure, increases in protein level and WBC, and CSF glucose lower than blood glucose)

(viii) Vascular disorders
1. Blood supply to the spinal cord depends on a single anterior spinal artery and bilateral posterior spinal arteries
2. Anterior spinal artery syndrome may result from arterial compression or hypotension
   (a) Characterized by a predominantly motor deficit, +/− loss of pain and temperature sensation, sparing of vibration and joint sensations
(ix) Cauda Equina
1. Risk factors:
   (a) Unintentional intrathecal injection of a large volume intended for the epidural space
   (b) Incorrect formulation with unsuitable preservative
   (c) Intrathecal lidocaine (especially hyperbaric 5%)
   (d) Repeat intrathecal injection for block failure
   (e) Fine-gauge or pencil-point needle
   (f) Spinal microcatheter
   (g) Continuous infusion
   (h) Hyperbaric anesthetic solution
   (i) Lithotomy position
(x) Transient Neurologic Syndrome
1. No detectable neurologic deficit
2. Characterized by pain in the back, buttocks, and thighs that mirrors the distribution of nerve damage in cauda equina
3. Risk factors are the same as cauda equine
4. Occurs four times more frequently with spinal lidocaine than with other local anesthetics.
(xi) Arachnoiditis – a disastrous condition with a delayed onset of permanent paraplegia
1. Seen after unintentional intrathecal injection of large doses of 2-chlorprocaine with antioxidant and preservative intended for epidural use.
2. Also seen with 2% lidocaine with preservative

Influence of Anesthetic Technique on Labor

24

1. Controversy exists as to whether neuraxial analgesia during labor is associated with a prolonged labor and operative delivery (i.e. cesarean delivery, forceps delivery, or vacuum extraction)
2. Women at higher risk for prolonged labor and operative delivery are more likely to request and receive epidural analgesia than women with a rapid, uncomplicated labor
   (a) Studies have shown higher levels of pain during the latent phase are predictive of longer latent and active phases of labor
   (b) These women were 2× as likely to require instrumental delivery
3. Epidurals placed before 4 cm dilation do not increase the rate of c-section
4. Epidurals have not been scientifically found to increase the rate of c-section
5. Instrumental vaginal delivery rates are increased in patients with epidurals because of dense epidurals causing motor blockade and/or because an OB is more likely to perform an elective instrumental delivery in a patient with satisfactory anesthesia than in one without
6. Neuraxial analgesia has a variable effect on the duration of the first stage of labor (shortens labor in some women and lengthens in others)
7. Effective neuraxial analgesia prolongs the second stage of labor by ~15–20 min
8. Neuraxial analgesia do not prolong the third stage of labor

© Springer Nature Switzerland AG 2019
C. Wasson et al., *Absolute Obstetric Anesthesia Review*,
https://doi.org/10.1007/978-3-319-96980-0_24

1. Indications
   (a) A prior cesarean delivery does not require a cesarean delivery in a subsequent pregnancy, except women at high risk of complication (e.g., those with previous classical or T-incision, prior uterine rupture, or extensive transfundal uterine surgery)
   (b) Maternal indications: antepartum or intrapartum hemorrhage; arrest of labor; breech presentation; chorioamnionitis; deteriorating maternal condition; dystocia; failure of induction of labor; active genital herpes; multiple gestation; maternal request; placenta previa; placental abruption; previous myomectomy; prior classic uterine incision; uterine rupture
   (c) Fetal indications: breech or other malpresentation; fetal intolerance of labor; macrosomia; non-reassuring FHT; prolapsed umbilical cord
   (d) OB indications: desire to avoid difficult forceps or vacuum delivery
2. Anesthetic techniques and complications
   (a) Neuraxial (e.g., spinal, epidural, CSE) – preferred method
       (i) Block needs to extend from sacral dermatomes to T4 because afferent nerves innervating abdominal and pelvic organs accompany sympathetic fibers that ascend and descend in the sympathetic trunk (T5-L1)
       (ii) Lower maternal morbidity and mortality compared to general anesthesia (GA)
       (iii) Decreased maternal blood loss and shivering than GA
       (iv) Increased maternal nausea than GA
       (v) Less post-op pain, GI stasis, coughing, fever, and depression than GA
       (vi) Recommended cocktail for spinal anesthesia for cesareans:
           1. Bupivacaine 12 mg (1.6 mL of 0.75%), fentanyl 10 mcg, and morphine 0.2 mg
       (vii) Local anesthetic and opioid doses are 5–10 times greater for epidurals than intrathecal
           1. Conversion of labor epidural to surgical epidural typically requires ~15–20 mL of local anesthetic with one or more adjuvants

© Springer Nature Switzerland AG 2019
C. Wasson et al., *Absolute Obstetric Anesthesia Review*,
https://doi.org/10.1007/978-3-319-96980-0_25

(b) General
- (i) Advantageous when uterine relaxation is beneficial (such as for Ex Utero Intrapartum Treatment (EXIT) procedures)
- (ii) Consent should feature risks associated with airway management, aspiration, and awareness
- (iii) Failed intubation, failed ventilation and oxygenation, and pulmonary aspiration of gastric contents are leading anesthesia-related causes of maternal death
- (iv) Desaturation occurs quicker due to decreased FRC and increased oxygen consumption during pregnancy
- (v) Patient's abdomen is prepped and draped prior to induction of GA to minimize fetal exposure to medications
- (vi) Rapid sequence induction (RSI) is required due to the increased risk of aspiration
- (vii) Thiopental (4–5 mg/kg) or propofol (2–2.8 mg/kg) are commonly used for induction
  1. Use ketamine (1–1.5 mg/kg) or etomidate (0.3 mg/kg) if hemodynamic instability is present
  2. Avoid ketamine in pre-eclampsia (further increases BP) and severe hypovolemia (can cause direct myocardial depression, decreased cardiac output, and hypotension in hypovolemic patients)
- (viii) Succinylcholine is used for paralysis
  1. Use rocuronium when succinylcholine is contraindicated (e.g., malignant hyperthermia, myotonic dystrophy, and spastic paraparesis)
  2. Remember, non-depolarizing muscle relaxants are enhanced by magnesium sulfate
- (ix) Use a smaller-diameter cuffed ETT
- (x) Normocapnia at term gestation is 30–32 mmHg
- (xi) Anesthetic requirements for volatiles are diminished 25–40% during pregnancy
- (xii) MAC > 1–1.5 may reduce the effect of oxytocin on uterine tone and increase blood loss
  1. Typically 1 MAC is administered between intubation and delivery
  2. MAC is often reduced to 0.5–0.75 after delivery. Nitrous oxide may help supplement as necessary to decrease the influence of volatiles on uterine tone
  3. Consider administering benzodiazepine (e.g. midazolam) after delivery to decrease risk of maternal awareness
- (xiii) Consider delayed extubation and/or transfer to ICU if repeated airway manipulation, massive hemorrhage, or emergency hysterectomy occurred

(c) Local
- (i) Used primarily in developing countries and to facilitate an emergency cesarean delivery
  1. Requires midline abdominal incision, avoiding use of retractors, and not exteriorizing the uterus
- (ii) Disadvantages: patient discomfort and potential for systemic local anesthetic toxicity
- (iii) Use of 0.5% lidocaine with epinephrine is recommended (total dose should not exceed 500 mg or 100 ml)

(d) Anesthetic complications
- (i) Awareness and recall
  1. Increased risk due to:
     (a) Avoidance of sedative premedications
     (b) The deliberate use of a low concentration of a volatile halogenated agent
     (c) The use of muscle relaxants
     (d) The reduction in dose of anesthetic agents during hypotension or hemorrhage
     (e) The presence of a partial neuraxial blockade in parturients requiring conversion to GA
     (f) The (mistaken) assumption that high baseline sympathetic tone is responsible for intraoperative tachycardia in parturients
  2. Administration of anxiolytic or hypnotic agents in patients receiving neuraxial technique may cause lack of recall of delivery, which is typically undesirable
- (ii) Dyspnea
  1. Follows administration of neuraxial technique
  2. Most common cause is hypotension causing hypoperfusion of the brainstem
     (a) Check BP and treat if needed
  3. Other causes:
     (a) Blunting of thoracic proprioception
     (b) Partial blockade of abdominal and intercostal muscles
     (c) Recumbent position (increased pressure of abdominal contents against diaphragm)
- (iii) Hypotension
  1. Common sequala of neuraxial anesthesia
  2. Fetal consequences: hypoxia, acidosis, and neonatal depression or injury
  3. Maternal consequences: unconsciousness, pulmonary aspiration, apnea, and cardiac arrest

(iv) Failure of neuraxial blockade
1. Neuroblockade insufficient in extent, density, or duration to provide anesthesia for c-section
2. Causes: anatomic, technical, and OB factors
3. Steps to reduce block failure:
   (a) Meticulous attention to technical detail
   (b) Administration of a solution that contains both a local anesthetic and an opioid
   (c) Better understanding of the characteristics of epidural versus spinal blockade
   (d) Educate the patient to expect the sensation of deep pressure and movement

(v) High neuraxial block
1. If impaired phonation, unconsciousness, respiratory depression, or significant impairment of ventilation occurs, administration of GA should be performed
2. Cardiovascular sequelae may occur (i.e., bradycardia and hypotension due to blockade of T1–4)

(vi) Nausea and vomiting
1. Very common with exteriorization of the uterus
2. Other causes: hypotension, increased vagal activity, surgical stimulus, bleeding, medications (e.g., uterotonic agents, antibiotics), and motion at the end of surgery
3. Preventing:
   (a) Preventing hypotension is the best means to prevent nausea and vomiting
   (b) Metoclopramide (prokinetic). Side effects: dizziness, drowsiness, and fatigue. May cause extrapyramidal reactions and acute dystonia
   (c) Ondansetron
   (d) Transdermal scopolamine. Side effects: dry mouth and blurry vision

(vii) Perioperative pain
1. Neuraxial morphine provides post-op analgesia
   (a) Peak effect at 60–90 min, but lasts up to 24 h
2. Postop pain may have at least two components: somatic and visceral

(viii) Pruritus
1. Treatment: opioid antagonist, opioid agonist/antagonist, droperidol, a serotonin antagonist (e.g., ondansetron), and/or a subhypnotic dose of propofol

(ix) Shivering may have several etiologies. Best treatment is meperidine
3. Difficult airway
   (a) Definition: difficulty placing an ETT via direct laryngoscopy or difficulty providing mask ventilation

(b) Higher risk of failed intubation in pregnancy due to airway edema, breast enlargement, obesity, and high rate of emergency surgery

  (i) Comorbid conditions are more common (due to delayed childbearing and use of assisted reproductive technologies), which may exacerbate the effects of hypoxemia, hypercarbia, and acidosis during delayed/failed intubation

(c) Airway edema can distort the anatomy of the larynx, decrease the size of the laryngeal opening, and necessitate use of smaller ETT

(d) If airway evaluation suggests possibility of difficult intubation in pre-op assessment, placement of a neuraxial catheter during early labor should be considered, even if it is not used to provide labor analgesia, in case patient requires cesarean

(e) Consider performing an awake endotracheal intubation

  (i) Oral fiberoptic larygoscopy is preferred because of the engorgement of the nasal mucosa and the potential for epistasis

  (ii) Administer antisialogogue (e.g., glycopyrrolate)

  (iii) Titrate benzodiazepine (e.g., midazolam) for sedation

  (iv) Use topical anesthesia in the upper airway with aerosolized lidocaine via standard nebulizer or an atomizer

  (v) Block glossopharyngeal nerve by bilateral administration of lidocaine just under the mucosa at the base of the anterior tonsillar pillars

  (vi) Block laryngeal sensation by blockade of the internal branch of the superior laryngeal nerve by bilateral injection of lidocaine at the thyro-hyoid membrane

    1. Alternative is to inject lidocaine through the fiberoptic side-port

(f) Options for failed endotracheal intubation

  (i) Awaken the patient

  (ii) Use alternative technique to intubate

  (iii) Use alternate airway device (e.g., LMA)

4. Aspiration prophylaxis

(a) Non-particulate antacids (e.g. sodium citrate) increases gastric pH, which decreases the risk of damage to the respiratory epithelium if aspiration should occur

(b) H2-receptor antagonists (ranitidine, famotidine) reduces secretion of gastric acid. Needs 30–40 min for effect.

(c) Metoclopramide is a promotility agent that hastens gastric emptying and also increases lower esophageal sphincter tone. It is also an antiemetic. Needs 30–40 min for effect. Dopamine antagonist centrally and cholinergic agonist peripherally.

  (i) Extrapyramidal effects are a major side effect

  (ii) Prior administration of an opioid or atropine antagonizes the effect of metoclopramide.

Part III

Pathophysiology of Complicated Pregnancy

Anesthesia for Cerclage

1. Performed for cervical insufficiency (recurrent second-trimester pregnancy losses with painless cervical dilation, herniation followed by rupture of fetal membranes, and short labor with delivery of live, immature infant)
2. Can be transvaginal or transabdominal
3. Performed prophylactically (before or during pregnancy), therapeutically (when cervical changes are noted in current pregnancy) or emergently (in patients with marked cervical changes including membrane exposure to vaginal environment)
4. Uterine relaxation is essential to replace bulging fetal membranes (administer volatile anesthetic or tocolytic) to decrease the risk of membrane rupture.
5. Transvaginal cervical cerclage can be performed under spinal, epidural, or general anesthesia.
   (a) The degree of cervical dilation may influence the choice of anesthesia.
   (b) GA with volatile anesthetics may be needed if the cervix is dilated and uterine relaxation is needed.
   (c) Sensory blockade from sacral dermatomes to T10 is necessary because both the cervix (L1 to T10) and vagina and perineum (S2–S4) require anesthesia

© Springer Nature Switzerland AG 2019
C. Wasson et al., *Absolute Obstetric Anesthesia Review*,
https://doi.org/10.1007/978-3-319-96980-0_26

Anesthesia for Non-obstetric Surgery

27

1. Risks to fetus: effects of the disease process itself or of related therapy, teratogenicity of anesthetic agents or other drugs administered during the perioperative period, intraoperative perturbations of uteroplacental perfusion and/or fetal oxygenation, and the risk of abortion or preterm delivery
2. Teratogenesis has not been associated with the commonly used induction agents (barbiturates, ketamine, and benzos), nor with opioids, local anesthetics, neuromuscular blockers, or volatile agents
3. Anesthesia and surgery are associated with a higher incidence of abortion, intrauterine growth restriction, and perinatal mortality. These adverse outcomes can be attributed to the procedure, the site of surgery (i.e. proximity to the uterus), and/or the underlying maternal condition. Evidence does not suggest anesthesia results in an increase in congenital abnormalities.
4. Fetal effects of anesthesia
    (a) Fetal hypoxemia due to maternal hypoxemia (due to difficult intubation, esophageal intubation, pulmonary aspiration, total spinal anesthesia, systemic local anesthetic toxicity)
    (b) Maternal hypercapnia causes fetal acidosis and subsequent myocardial depression and hypotension
    (c) Maternal hyperventilation/hypocapnia leads to umbilical artery constriction and left shift of maternal oxyhemoglobin dissociation curve, which decreases maternal-fetal oxygen transfer
    (d) Maternal hypotension decreases uteroplacental perfusion
    (e) Minimal fetal effects are seen at 1 MAC of volatiles; decreased uteroplacental perfusion with 2 MAC
5. Risk of preterm labor is lowest during second trimester, therefore this is the optimal period to have nonobstetric surgery without risk of teratogenicity and preterm labor.

© Springer Nature Switzerland AG 2019
C. Wasson et al., *Absolute Obstetric Anesthesia Review*,
https://doi.org/10.1007/978-3-319-96980-0_27

6. Preop management
    (a) Premedication for anxiolysis may be necessary
    (b) Pregnancy increases risk of acid aspiration after 18–20 weeks' gestation. Pre-medicate with H2 antagonist, metoclopramide, or a clear non-particulate antacid (i.e. sodium citrate)
7. Local or regional anesthesia is preferred when possible
8. Patient should be placed with left lateral tilt to prevent aortocaval compression
9. Fetal heart rate and uterine activity should be monitored before and after surgery. Intra-op monitoring on a case-by-case basis
10. Avoid: hypotension, hypoxemia, acidosis, and hyper- and hypocapnia

28

1. Fertilized ovum implants outside the endometrial lining of the uterus
2. Ruptured ectopic is leading cause of pregnancy-related maternal death during first trimester
   (a) Due to hemorrhage (93%), infection (2.5%), embolism (2.1%), and anesthetic complications (1.3%)
3. Increased risk of ectopic in:
   (a) Prior ectopic pregnancy
   (b) Prior tubal surgery
   (c) Pelvic inflammation (especially Chlamydia infection)
   (d) Congenital anatomic distortions, such as that caused by diethylstilbestrol (DES) in utero
   (e) Previous pelvic or abdominal surgery
   (f) Use of IUD
   (g) Delayed ovulation
   (h) Hormonal changes associated with ovulation induction or progestin-only oral contraceptives
   (i) Lifestyle choices (e.g. smoking, vaginal douching)
   (j) History of infertility
   (k) Assisted reproductive technology procedures
4. Location of ectopic: tubal (98%) (78% ampullary, 12% isthmic, 6% infundibular/fimbrial, 2% interstitial/cornual), remaining 2% are abdominal, cervical, vaginal, or ovarian
5. Clinical signs/symptoms: abdominal/pelvic pain, delayed menses, and vaginal bleeding
6. Diagnosis:
   (a) Ultrasonography: transvaginal preferred as can detect intrauterine gestational sac sooner than transabdominal
   (b) Serial beta-hCG concentrations that decrease, plateau, or show a subnormal rise
      (i) Decline of 21–35% over 2 days suggests spontaneous abortion, slower decline is suggestive of ectopic

© Springer Nature Switzerland AG 2019
C. Wasson et al., *Absolute Obstetric Anesthesia Review*,
https://doi.org/10.1007/978-3-319-96980-0_28

7. Obstetric management:
   (a) Expectant management
       (i) Used for asymptomatic patients with early tubal ectopic pregnancies
       (ii) Successful resolution occurs in 50% of patients
   (b) Medical management
       (i) Systemic, intramuscular, oral, or intragestational forms of chemotherapy (typically methotrexate)
   (c) Surgical management
       (i) Diagnostic laparoscopy utilized to confirm diagnosis and locate ectopic pregnancy
       (ii) Tubal ectopics undergo salpingostomy, salpingotomy, or salpingectomy
   (d) Patients with ectopic pregnancies who are Rh negative should receive Rho(D) immune globulin

Spontaneous Abortion

29

1. Occurs before 20 weeks' gestation or when fetus weighs <500 g
2. Etiology: chromosomal (50–80%), remainder are immunologic mechanisms, maternal infections, endocrine abnormalities (e.g. poorly controlled DM), uterine anomalies, incompetent cervix, debilitating maternal disease, trauma, and possibly environmental exposures (e.g. irradiation, smoking, certain drugs)
3. Threatened abortion: uterine bleeding without cervical dilation <20 weeks gestation
4. Inevitable abortion: cervical dilation or rupture of membranes without expulsion of fetus or placenta
5. Complete abortion: total, spontaneous rupture of fetus and placenta
6. Incomplete abortion: partial expulsion of uterine contents
7. Rh negative mothers must receive Rho(D) immune globulin to prevent Rh sensitization

© Springer Nature Switzerland AG 2019
C. Wasson et al., *Absolute Obstetric Anesthesia Review*,
https://doi.org/10.1007/978-3-319-96980-0_29

Gestational Trophoblastic Disease (Hydatidiform Mole)

30

1. Complete hydatidiform moles (90% of hydatid moles) are derived solely from paternal chromosomes (ovum lacking maternal chromosomal complement is fertilized by one sperm (46,XX androgenic) or by two sperm (dispermy 46,XX or 46,XY androgenic))
   (a) No fetus develops
2. Partial moles have complete trisomy (69,XXX or 69,XXY) (one set of chromosomes are maternal and two sets are paternal)
   (a) Often associated with fetal tissue
3. Clinical diagnosis: vaginal bleeding after delayed menses (as seen in threatened, missed, or incomplete abortion)
4. Hydatidiform moles have uterus large for gestational age, markedly elevated beta-hCG and lack of fetal cardiac activity
5. These patients are more prone to hyperemesis gravidarum, pregnancy-induced hypertension (PIH), severe anemia, and/or hyperthyroidism (the alpha subunit of hCG is structurally similar to thyroid stimulating hormone (TSH))
6. Signs and symptoms of acute cardiopulmonary distress develop after uterine evacuation in as many as 27% of molar pregnancies

© Springer Nature Switzerland AG 2019
C. Wasson et al., *Absolute Obstetric Anesthesia Review*,
https://doi.org/10.1007/978-3-319-96980-0_30

Autoimmune Disorders

31

1. Systemic lupus erythematos
   - (a) Antibodies against nuclear, cytoplasmic, and cell membrane antigens
   - (b) Diagnosis requires 4+ symptoms:
       - (i) Malar rash (butterfly rash)
       - (ii) Discoid rash (erythematous, raised patches with scaling)
       - (iii) Photosensitivity
       - (iv) Oral ulceration
       - (v) Arthritis
       - (vi) Serositis (pleuritis or pericarditis)
       - (vii) Renal disorder (persistent proteinuria or cellular casts)
       - (viii) Neurologic disorder (seizures or psychosis)
       - (ix) Hematologic disorder (hemolytic anemia, leukopenia, lymphopenia, or thrombocytopenia)
       - (x) Immunologic disorder (anti-DNA, anti-SM nuclear antigen, anticardiolipin antibodies, lupus anticoagulant, or false-positive syphilis test)
       - (xi) Antinuclear antibody
   - (c) Neonatal lupus erythematosus is a syndrome that may result when maternal autoantibodies against Ro (SS-A) or La (SS-B) cross the placenta and bind to fetal tissue
       - (i) **Reversible** manifestations (i.e., cutaneous lupus, transaminase elevation, and thrombocytopenia) resolve when maternal antibodies disappear from the newborn circulation (within 8 months after birth)
       - (ii) These antibodies may also bind to conduction cells during fetal cardiac conduction system development leading to **irreversible** fetal heart block.
   - (d) Medications
       - (i) Continue hydroxychloroquinine to decrease risk of increased disease activity
       - (ii) Continue azathioprine

© Springer Nature Switzerland AG 2019
C. Wasson et al., *Absolute Obstetric Anesthesia Review*,
https://doi.org/10.1007/978-3-319-96980-0_31

   (iii) Mycophenolate mofetil is teratogenic, so needs to be discontinued prior to conception (azathioprine is a substitute)

   (iv) Low-dose prednisone is safe, but other corticosteroids (e.g., dexamethasone or betamethasone) may lead to decreased intrauterine growth and abnormal neuronal development

  (e) Increased risk of preterm delivery and intrauterine fetal death

  (f) These patients may have autoantibodies against specific coagulation factors (e.g., VIII, IX, XII) contraindicating neuraxial anesthesia

2. Antiphospholipid syndrome

  (a) Prothrombotic disorder causing both arterial and venous thrombosis

  (b) Two antibodies: lupus anticoagulant and anticardiolipin antibody

  (c) High risk for recurrent pregnancy loss, likely due to placental infarct

  (d) These patients are prescribed low-dose aspirin and prophylactic heparin during pregnancy and for 6–8 weeks postpartum

   (i) If history of thrombosis, patients receive full anticoagulation throughout pregnancy and postpartum

3. Systemic sclerosis (scleroderma)

  (a) Deposition of fibrous connective tissue in the skin and other tissues

  (b) Autoantibodies to nuclear and centromere structures

  (c) Diagnosed by triad of Raynaud's phenomenon, non-pitting edema, and hidebound skin

  (d) Two types: limited cutaneous scleroderma and diffuse cutaneous scleroderma

   (i) Limited cutaneous scleroderma (AKA CREST syndrome): calcinosis, Raynaud's phenomenon, esophageal dysfunction, sclerodactyly, and telangiectasia

   (ii) Diffuse cutaneous scleroderma involves multiple systems:

    1. Skin: Raynaud's phenomenon, non-pitting edema, Hidebound skin

    2. GI: hypomotility, dysphagia, reflux esophagitis, postprandial fullness, constipation, abdominal pain, intermittent diarrhea, malnutrition, ileus

    3. Pulmonary: interstitial fibrosis, pleuritic, pulmonary hypertension

    4. Renal: proteinuria, renal insufficiency and failure, malignant hypertension

    5. Cardiac: chronic pericardial effusion, myocardial ischemia and infarction, conduction disturbances, heart failure

    6. Musculoskeletal: arthritis (symmetric, small joints), myopathy, muscle wasting

    7. Other: peripheral or cranial neuropathy, facial pain, trigeminal neuralgia, keratoconjunctivitis sicca, xerostomia, and absence of anti-centromere antibodies

  (e) Increased risk of preterm birth, mainly in women with unstable diffuse scleroderma

  (f) No treatment exists. Therapy is directed toward symptom management

(g) Patient may have severe limitation of the oral opening from perioral hide-bound skin, making direct laryngoscopy impossible

(h) These patients may have prolonged duration of regional anesthesia, likely due to microvasculature changes that diminish uptake of the local anesthetic agent

4. Polymyositis and dermatomyositis – idiopathic inflammatory myopathic diseases

   (a) Polymyositis – nonsuppurative inflammation of muscle

       (i) Leads to symmetric weakness, atrophy, and fibrosis

       (ii) Primarily skeletal muscles of the proximal limbs, neck and pharynx

           1. Pharyngeal muscle involvement leads to dysphagia and reflux

           2. Chronic aspiration pneumonitis is common

           3. Myositis of the respiratory muscles may cause respiratory insufficiency

           4. Cardiac involvement includes nonspecific repolarization abnormalities, conduction disturbances, arrhythmias, coronary artery vasculitis, and, rarely, heart failure

   (b) Dermatomyositis is polymyositis with the addition of characteristic heliotrope eruption (blue-purple discoloration of the upper eyelid) and Gottron's papules (raised, scaly, violet eruptions over the knuckles)

   (c) Etiology is unknown.

   (d) Associated with other autoimmune disorders, notably scleroderma

   (e) Diagnostic criteria

       (i) Polymyositis

           1. Symmetric weakness of proximal muscles

           2. Histologic evidence of muscle inflammation and necrosis on muscle biopsy

           3. Elevation of serum skeletal muscle enzymes

           4. Electromyographic evidence of myopathy

       (ii) Dermatomyositis

           1. Three or four of the polymyositis criteria, plus heliotrope eruptions or Gottron's papules

   (f) Active disease often ends in fetal death or spontaneous abortion

   (g) Uneventful outcomes of pregnancy if disease is in remission

   (h) Medical management of active disease is glucocorticoids

Diabetes Mellitus (DM)

1. Caused by a deficiency in insulin secretion (type I) or a combination of resistance to insulin in target tissues and inadequate insulin secretion (type II)
2. Acute and chronic complications occur in patients with DM
   (a) Three major acute complications: DKA, hyperglycemic nonketotic state, and hypoglycemia
   (b) Chronic complications (decreased risk with tight glucose control):
      (i) Macrovascular (atherosclerosis): coronary, cerebrovascular, and peripheral vascular
      (ii) Microvascular: retinopathy and nephropathy
      (iii) Neuropathy: autonomic and somatic
3. Gestational DM – DM or glucose intolerance first diagnosed during pregnancy
   (a) Associated with: advanced maternal age; obesity; family history of type 2 DM; prior history of gestational DM; history of PCOS; glycosuria; and/or history of prior stillbirth, neonatal death, fetal malformation, or macrosomia
   (b) Pregnancy has a progressive peripheral resistance to insulin at the receptor and post-receptor levels in the second and third trimesters
      (i) Presumed mechanism is an increase in counter-regulatory hormones (e.g., placental lactogen, placental growth hormone, cortisol, progesterone)
4. Beta-adrenergic receptor agonists (to treat preterm labor) and corticosteroids (to accelerate fetal lung maturity) can precipitate DKA in pregnancy due to pharmacologic opposition of insulin
5. Pre-gestational type I diabetics are three times as likely as nondiabetic patients to have gestational HTN
   (a) Risk of preeclampsia is increased with increased severity of diabetes (determined by duration of diabetes and any concurrent diabetic chronic complications (e.g., nephropathy, neuropathy, retinopathy, etc))
6. Pregestational and gestational DM has higher rates of gestational HTN, polyhydramnios and cesarean delivery

© Springer Nature Switzerland AG 2019
C. Wasson et al., *Absolute Obstetric Anesthesia Review*,
https://doi.org/10.1007/978-3-319-96980-0_32

7. Pregestational DM (NOT gestational DM) is associated with a 2–3× increased incidence of preterm labor and delivery
8. Fetal complications of maternal DM
   (a) During pregnancy
      (i) Chronic
         1. Macrosomia
            (a) Shoulder dystocia
            (b) Birth injury or trauma
         2. Structural malformations
            (a) CNS (meningomyelocele, anencephaly, encephalocele, spina bifida, holoprosencephaly)
            (b) Cardiac (transposition of the great vessels, VSD, situs inversus, single ventricle, hypoplastic left ventricle)
            (c) Skeletal (caudal regression)
            (d) Renal (agenesis, multicystic dysplasia)
            (e) Gastrointestinal (anal or rectal atresia, small left colon)
         3. Pulmonary (hypoplasia)
      (ii) Acute
         1. Intrauterine or neonatal death
         2. Neonatal RDS
         3. Neonatal hypoglycemia
         4. Neonatal hyperbilirubinemia
   (b) Post-pregnancy
      (iii) Glucose intolerance
      (iv) Possible impairment of cognitive development
   (c) Of the fetal anomalies, cardiac anomalies are the most common, followed by CNS
   (d) Strict glycemic control prior to conception in patients with pregesional DM:
      (v) reduces the rate of major congenital anomalies from 10% to 1% (the same as that of the general population)
      (vi) decreases the rate of spontaneous abortions
9. Diabetic stiff-joint syndrome (AKA diabetic scleroderma) is associated with difficult DL and intubation in patients with DM
   (a) Occurs in long-standing DMI patients and causes limited movement of the AO joint
   (b) Can be screened for by looking for the "prayer sign"
   (c) Figure 32.1: Prayer sign
   (d) In patients with H&P suggestive of diabetic stiff-joint syndrome, anesthesia providers should consider two potential problems: difficult DL/intubation and a noncompliant epidural space

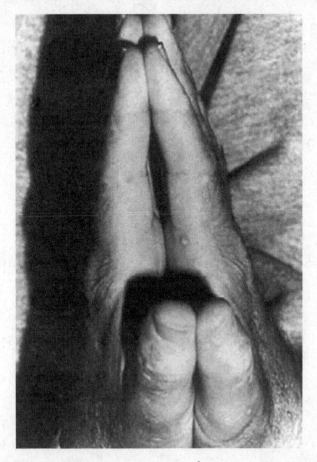

Fig. 32.1 Inability to approximate the palmar surfaces of the phalangeal joints despite maximal effort, secondary to diabetic stiff-joint syndrome. (From Hogan K, Rusy D, Springman SR. Difficult laryngoscopy and diabetes mellitus. *Anesth Analg* 1988;67:1162–5)

Thyroid Disorders

33

1. During normal pregnancy, the serum concentration of thyroxine-binding globulin (TBG) steadily increases until it reaches a plateau at 20 weeks' gestation due to a prolonged half-life (not higher synthesis) during pregnancy. The rise in TBG leads to an increase in both serum total, but not free, T4 and T3 concentrations
2. Hyperthyroidism
   (a) Etiologies
      (i) Abnormal thyroid stimulator (e.g., Graves' disease, gestational trophoblastic neoplasia, or Thyroid-stimulating hormone-secreting pituitary tumor)
         1. Graves' (autoimmune thyroid disease) is the most common cause and accounts for 70–90% of cases
         2. Gestational trophoblastic neoplasms are often associated with elevated serum hCG, which mimics TSH
      (ii) Intrinsic thyroid autonomy (e.g., toxic adenoma or toxic multinodular goiter)
      (iii) Inflammatory disease (i.e. subacute thyroiditis)
      (iv) Extrinsic hormone source (e.g., ectopic thyroid tissue or thyroid hormone ingestion)
   (b) Treatment:
      (i) Radioactive iodine: typically leads to hypothyroidism after therapeutic dose. It is contraindicated in pregnancy
      (ii) Propylthiouracil and methimazole are antithyroid medications to treat Graves'. Major complication is asymptomatic agranulocytosis.
         1. Both reduce thyroid hormone production
         2. Only PTU inhibits peripheral conversion of T_4 to T_3
         3. PTU is safe in pregnancy
      (iii) Surgical therapy: in Graves', it is reserved for those unable or unwilling to do pharmacologic treatment or who have failed treatment
         1. Periop complications: unilateral or bilateral vocal cord paralysis due to laryngeal nerve injury; wound hematoma; pneumothorax; hypoparathyroidism (and subsequent hypocalcemia); and thyroid storm

© Springer Nature Switzerland AG 2019
C. Wasson et al., *Absolute Obstetric Anesthesia Review*,
https://doi.org/10.1007/978-3-319-96980-0_33

      (iv) Adjunctive therapies include iodine, lithium, radiocontrast agents, and glucocorticoids

      (v) Beta blockers are used to decreased CV response

        1. Propranolol is the beta blocker of choice as also inhibits peripheral conversion of T_4 to T_3

        2. May increase the risk of preterm labor

(c) Poorly controlled hyperthyroidism during pregnancy increases the risk of severe preeclampsia in the mother and low birth weight in the neonate

(d) In women with Graves' disease, the placental transfer of anti-thyroid medications or thyroid-stimulating Ab may result in the development of fetal goiter, which can interfere with vaginal delivery or lead to airway obstruction in the neonate

(e) Features of hyperthyroidism that may affect anesthetic management: hyperdynamic CV system and possibility of cardiomyopathy; partial airway obstruction from enlarged thyroid gland; respiratory muscle weakness; and electrolyte abnormalities

3. Hypothyroidism

  (a) Causes:

    (i) Primary

      1. Autoimmune (e.g., Hashimoto's thyroiditis and atrophic hypothyroidism)

      2. Iatrogenic (radioiodine therapy for hyperthyroidism and subtotal thyroidectomy)

      3. Pharmacologic (iodine deficiency or excess, lithium, amiodarone, and antithyroid drugs)

      4. Congenital (Dyshormonogenesis, thyroid gland dysgenesis or agenesis)

    (ii) Secondary

      1. Pituitary dysfunction (irradiation, surgery, neoplasm, Sheehan's syndrome, idiopathic)

      2. Hypothalamic dysfunction (irradiation, granulomatous disease, neoplasm)

  (b) Treated with levothyroxine; dose needs to be increased during pregnancy

  (c) Increased incidence of anemia, preeclampsia, IUGR, placental abruption, and postpartum hemorrhage

  (d) Features of hypothyroidism that may affect anesthetic management: reversible myocardial dysfunction; CAD; reversible defects in hypoxic and hypercapnic ventilatory drives; OSA; paresthesias; prolonged SSEP central conduction time; increased CSF protein concentrations; increased peripheral nociceptive thresholds; hyponatremia; decreased glucocorticoid reserves; anemia; and abnormal coagulation factors and platelets

  (e) Hypothyroidism is a rare cause of acquired von Willebrand's disease

  (f) Use findings from the H&P and lab testing to verify normal coagulation prior to administering neuraxial anesthesia in untreated hypothyroid patients

Pheochromocytoma

34

1. Pheochromocytoma – Tumor of chromaffin cells of neuroectodermal origin that secretes norepinephrine and epinephrine
2. Rare during pregnancy
3. 90% are in the medulla of one or both adrenal glands
4. Bilateral in 10% of cases; malignant in 10% of cases
5. Part of MEN2A (medullary thyroid carcinoma, hyperparathyroidism, pheochromocytoma) and MEN2B (medullary thyroid carcinoma, mucocutaneous neuromas, pheochromocytoma)
6. Other disease processes associated with pheochromocytoma: von Recklinghausen's, von Hippel-Lindau, Sturge-Weber, and tuberous sclerosis
7. Hypertension is common, but not universal (paroxysmal is more common than sustained)
8. Orthostatic hypotension occurs in 70% of pheochromocytoma
9. Diagnosis involves three steps:
   (a) Biochemical testing for increased catecholamine secretion
      (i) Measure norepinephrine or epinephrine or concentrations of their metabolites (normetanephrine, metanephrine, or vanillylmandelic acid) in plasma or urine
   (b) Anatomic imaging
   (c) Functional imaging
      (i) Meta-iodobenzylguanidine (MIBG) is used for scintigraphic localization
      (ii) PET with fluorine-18-L-dihydroxyphenylalanine can also be used, but is less available
10. Definitive treatment is surgical resection
   (a) Severe hypertension may occur during induction of anesthesia and surgical manipulation of the tumor
   (b) Severe hypotension frequently occurs after excision

C. Wasson et al., *Absolute Obstetric Anesthesia Review*,
https://doi.org/10.1007/978-3-319-96980-0_34

11. Preoperative preparation includes alpha-blockers and IV volume repletion
    (a) Most commonly used alpha-blocker is phenoxybenzamine
        (i) Doxazosin, prazosin, and phentolamine have also been used successfully
    (b) Beta-blockers may be added to treat arrhythmias, but must not be used prior to alpha-blockade to prevent paradoxical hypertensive response
12. Intra-op management
    (a) Treat episodic hypertension and tachycardia prior to excision with short acting agents: nitroprusside, nitroglycerin, esmolol, magnesium sulfate, and adenosine
    (b) Treat profound hypotension after excision
    (c) Hypoglycemia may occur after resection as insulin secretion is inhibited by alpha-adrenergic receptor stimulation, and removal of the tumor may result in rebound of insulin release. Blood glucose should be measured frequently after tumor excision
13. Management during pregnancy
    (a) Open or laparoscopic tumor resection at 16–21 weeks' gestation (after patient is adequately adrenergically blocked) followed by vaginal delivery at term
    (b) After 24 weeks' gestation, patient should receive adrenergic blockade (alpha blockers and beta-blockers have been used safely during pregnancy) for the remainder of the pregnancy and until tumor is removed and undergo one of the following options:
        (i) Cesarean delivery with concurrent open tumor resection
        (ii) Cesarean delivery with open or laparoscopic tumor resection 2–8 weeks later
        (iii) Vaginal delivery with laparoscopic tumor resection 6 weeks later
    (c) Nitroprusside should be used with caution in pregnancy due to concern of fetal cyanide toxicity. Low dose (~1 µg/kg/min) should be safe during the peripartum period.
        (i) If maternal tachyphylaxis develops, it should be discontinued and another vasodilator used
14. Untreated pheochromocytoma during pregnancy increases the rate of fetal death and IUGR
    (a) Placental abruption can occur
    (b) May be misdiagnosed as preeclampsia
    (c) Cesarean delivery is preferred to vaginal to avoid increased abdominal pressure on the tumor during labor
15. Spinal and epidural anesthesia have both been used successfully

16. Medications to avoid during anesthesia in pheochromocytoma because they can
    precipitate severe hypertension:
    (a) Dopamine-blocking drugs: metoclopramide, droperidol, haloperidol
    (b) Glucagon (can release catecholamines from tumors)
    (c) Sympathomimetic drugs: ketamine, cocaine, ephedrine, pancuronium, suc-
        cinylcholine (fasciculation of abdominal muscles can increase catechol-
        amine release from tumor mass)
    (d) Histamine-releasing medications: morphine, atracurium, cisatracurium,
        mivacurium

Congenital Heart Disease

35

1. Congenital heart disease represent 60–80% of cardiac disease in pregnant women
2. Left-to-right shunts (i.e., ASD, VSD, PDA)
   (a) ASD complications: arrhythmias, pulmonary HTN, and right ventricle (RV) failure; complications usually develop after age 40
   (b) VSD and PDA typically close spontaneously or are surgically repaired in childhood
   (c) Anesthetic management
      (i) Avoid IV infusion of air bubbles and use of loss-of-resistance to saline (rather than air) to identify the epidural space
      (ii) Minimize pain-associated increases in maternal plasma catecholamine concentrations and SVR
      (iii) Gradual onset of sympathetic blockade avoids a abrupt decrease in SVR, which can cause a L-to-R shunt to become a R-to-L shunt with subsequent hypoxemia
      (iv) Avoid pain, hypoxemia, hypercarbia, and acidosis, which can increase pulmonary vascular resistance and reverse the shunt flow
3. Coarctation of the aorta
   (a) High risk for LV failure, aortic rupture or dissection, and endocarditis
      (i) Fetal mortality rate is approximately 20% due to reduced uteroplacental perfusion distal to the aortic lesion
   (b) These patients are higher risk for bicuspid aortic valves (and increased risk of endocarditis) or aneurysms of the circle of Willis
      (i) Labor increases the risk of intracranial aneurysm rupture or aortic dissection due to wide fluctuations in BP, so many OBs recommend elective cesarean delivery
   (c) If coarctation was surgically corrected, or arm-to-leg BP gradient is <20 mmHg, vaginal delivery is preferred

© Springer Nature Switzerland AG 2019
C. Wasson et al., *Absolute Obstetric Anesthesia Review*,
https://doi.org/10.1007/978-3-319-96980-0_35

4. Tetralogy of Fallot
   (a) Represent 5% of cases of congenital heart disease in pregnant women
   (b) Four components: VSD, RV hypertrophy, pulmonic stenosis with RV out-
       flow tract obstruction, and overriding aorta
   (c) Most have surgical correction in childhood
   (d) Cardiovascular changes of pregnancy (i.e., increased blood volume and CO,
       and reduced SVR) may unmask previously asymptomatic residua of cor-
       rected tetralogy
   (e) Anesthetic management in corrected lesions is no different than in patients
       without this lesion
   (f) For parturients with uncorrected tetralogy or corrected with residua, avoid
       decreases in SVR (worsens the severity of R-to-L shunt) and maintain ade-
       quate intravascular volume and venous return
       (i) Single-shot spinal is poor choice for cesarean delivery due to abrupt
           reduction in SVR. Epidural with slow titration is preferred
5. Eisenmenger's Syndrome
   (a) Uncorrected L-to-R shunt leading to RV hypertrophy, elevated pulmonary
       artery pressures, RV dysfunction
   (b) Most common cause: VSD, followed by PDA, and less commonly ASD
   (c) The drop in SVR associated with pregnancy exacerbates the R-to-L shunt,
       leading to worsening hypoxemia
       (i) Hypoxemia causes high incidence of intrauterine growth restriction and
           fetal demise
   (d) Anesthetic goals:
       (i) Maintain SVR
       (ii) Maintain intravascular volume and venous return
       (iii) Avoid aortocaval compression
       (iv) Prevent pain, hypoxia, hypercarbia, and acidosis (worsens pulmonary
            vascular resistance)
       (v) Avoid myocardial depression during GA

Valvular Disorders

36

1. Aortic stenosis
   (a) Lesions become hemodynamically significant when the valve diameter is one third of its normal size
      (i) Severe aortic stenosis is a valve area <0.8–1.0 cm^2 and a peak gradient >40–50 mmHg
   (b) Asymptomatic aortic stenosis tolerate pregnancy well
   (c) Women with severe aortic stenosis are advised to have corrective surgery before conception as they are unable to compensate for the greater demands of pregnancy
   (d) Vaginal delivery is preferred mode of delivery
   (e) Anesthetic management: maintain normal heart rate, sinus rhythm, and adequate SVR; maintain intravascular volume and venous return; avoid aortocaval compression; avoid myocardial depression during GA
2. Aortic regurgitation
   (a) More common than aortic stenosis in women of childbearing age
   (b) Typically tolerates pregnancy well
   (c) Goals of anesthetic management: maintain normal to slightly elevated HR; prevent an increase in SVR; avoid aortocaval compression; avoid myocardial depression during GA
3. Mitral stenosis
   (a) Most common valvular lesion in pregnancy
   (b) Mild stenosis is valve area >1.5 cm^2; moderate is 1–1.5 cm^2; severe is <1 cm^2
   (c) Women with severe mitral stenosis do not tolerate the cardiovascular demands of pregnancy
   (d) Associated with atrial fibrillation
   (e) Anticoagulation to prevent systemic embolization

© Springer Nature Switzerland AG 2019
C. Wasson et al., *Absolute Obstetric Anesthesia Review*,
https://doi.org/10.1007/978-3-319-96980-0_36

   (f) Anesthetic goals: maintain slow heart rate and sinus rhythm; treat acute atrial fibrillation aggressively; avoid aortocaval compression; maintain adequate venous return; maintain adequate SVR; and prevent pain, hypoxemia, hypercarbia, and acidosis, which may increase pulmonary vascular resistance

4. Mitral regurgitation
   (a) Hemodynamic changes of pregnancy are beneficial for mitral regurgitation due to the lower SVR promoting forward flow
   (b) Anticoagulation indicated in concomitant atrial fibrillation
   (c) Anesthetic goals: prevent increases in SVR; maintain normal to slightly increased heart rate in sinus rhythm; aggressively treat acute atrial fibrillation; avoid aortocaval compression; maintain venous return; prevent increases in central vascular volume; avoid myocardial depression during GA; and prevent pain, hypoxemia, hypercarbia, and acidosis, which may increase pulmonary vascular resistance

5. Mitral valve prolapse
   (a) Most common cardiac condition encountered during pregnancy
   (b) These women generally tolerate pregnancy well
   (c) Neuraxial analgesia is an excellent choice for labor and vaginal or cesarean delivery; the sympathectomy and decreased catecholamines are beneficial

6. Prior prosthetic valve surgery
   (a) Patients with mechanical heart valves must maintain anticoagulation during pregnancy
     (i) Warfarin crosses the placenta and is associated with a higher incidence of spontaneous abortion, preterm delivery, intrauterine fetal death, and fetal bleeding
     (ii) Heparin does not cross the placenta, so is the anticoagulant of choice
   (b) Normal or near-normal coagulation parameters and adequate platelet count should be present before administration of neuraxial anesthesia and prior to removal of epidural or spinal catheter

7. Cardiac surgery during pregnancy
   (a) High pump flow rates (>2.5 L/min/m^2) and high MAP (>70 mmHg) are recommended to optimize uteroplacental perfusion

Other Heart Disease

37

1. Primary pulmonary hypertension – elevated pulmonary artery pressures in the absence of an intracardiac or aortopulmonary shunt
   (a) Pregnancy and delivery are poorly tolerated
   (b) High incidence of IUGR, fetal loss, and preterm labor
   (c) Anesthetic goals are same as Eisenmenger's syndrome (see above)
   (d) O_2 is a pulmonary vasodilator and should be administered routinely to these patients
2. Hypertrophic obstructive cardiomyopathy (HOCM)
   (a) Cardiomyopathy affecting the interventricular septum in the area of the LV outflow tract
   (b) Characteristics: LV hypertrophy, decreased LV chamber size, and LV dysfunction
   (c) Management: slow heart rate and modest expansion of intravascular volume
   (d) Avoid increases in myocardial contractility and decreases in SVR (these exacerbate degree of outflow tract obstruction)
   (e) Increased risk of sudden death from ventricular arrhythmias
   (f) Higher risk of maternal mortality than in the general population, but absolute risk of maternal mortality is low
   (g) Tolerate vaginal delivery well
   (h) Anesthetic goals:
       (i) Maintain intravascular volume and venous return
       (ii) Avoid aortocaval compression
       (iii) Maintain adequate SVR
       (iv) Maintain slow heart rate in sinus rhythm
       (v) Aggressive treatment of acute atrial fibrillation and other tachyarrhythmias
       (vi) Prevention of increases in myocardial contractility
   (i) Relative contraindication to single-shot spinal due to rapid onset of sympathectomy

© Springer Nature Switzerland AG 2019
C. Wasson et al., *Absolute Obstetric Anesthesia Review*,
https://doi.org/10.1007/978-3-319-96980-0_37

3. Ischemic heart disease
   (a) Incidence is increasing due to:
       (i) Delayed and extended childbearing (pregnancies in 5th, 6th, 7th decades of life due to embryo donation)
       (ii) Continued use of tobacco
       (iii) Cocaine abuse
       (iv) Oral contraceptive use after age 35
   (b) Risk factors: HTN, DM, thrombophilia, smoking, age greater than 35, and black race
       (i) OB risk factors: preeclampsia, postpartum hemorrhage, and the requirement of a blood transfusion.
   (c) Abnormal EKG findings that are normal in pregnancy: sinus tachycardia, leftward axis shift, ST-segment depression, flattened or inverted T waves, and a Q wave in lead III
   (d) Anesthetic management for ischemic heart disease
       (i) Supplemental O_2 during labor and delivery
       (ii) Epidural analgesia throughout labor to minimize hyperdynamic circulatory changes
4. Peripartum cardiomyopathy
   (a) Etiology is unknown
   (b) Diagnosis is made with the following three criteria:
       (i) Heart failure develops in the last month of pregnancy or within 5 months of delivery
       (ii) EF < 45%
       (iii) No other cause for heart failure with reduced EF
   (c) Supportive/symptomatic management
5. Arrhythmias
   (a) Increased frequency in pregnancy, most common being premature atrial contractions and premature ventricular contractions
   (b) Fetus is at increased risk for preterm delivery, small for gestational age, fetal demise, respiratory distress syndrome, and intraventricular hemorrhage
   (c) Antiarrhythmic medications
       (i) Digitalis – treats maternal atrial tachyarrhythmias. Crosses the placenta, but does not affect neonatal EKG
       (ii) Quinidine – treats atrial tachyarrhythmias. No evidence of teratogenicity. Associated with preterm labor
       (iii) Beta-blockers – variety of indications (i.e., HTN, mitral stenosis, HOCM, and control of heart rate in atrial and ventricular tachyarrhythmias). Cross the placenta and cause IUGR, fetal bradycardia, and neonatal hypoglycemia.
       (iv) Calcium channel blockers – verapamil crosses the placenta and may slow the AV conduction in the fetus. Nicardipine is often used to treat severe preeclampsia
       (v) Lidocaine – treats ectopic ventricular arrhythmias during pregnancy. Fetal acidosis may result in ion trapping

(vi) Amiodarone – adverse fetal effects including IUGR, preterm delivery, and fetal hypothyroidism. Treats refractory maternal atrial and ventricular arrhythmias, as well as fetal tachyarrhythmias.

(vii) Adenosine – agent of choice for acute management of tachyarrhythmias. Unlikely to affect fetus due to short half-life.

(d) Patient with congenital heart block may be asymptomatic until pregnancy.

   (i) If become symptomatic in the first or second trimester, permanent pacemaker implantation is the therapy of choice.

   (ii) If the patient is at or near term, temporary pacing immediately before the induction of labor is the treatment of choice. Reassess the patient in the postpartum period to determine if implantation of a permanent pacemaker is warranted.

(e) Prolonged QT increases the risk for torsades de pointes and cardiac arrest during pregnancy

   (i) Beta-blockers are mainstay of treatment

   (ii) Cardiac pacing may be required for patients unresponsive to beta-blockers

   (iii) Critical episodes may be treated with cardioversion or defibrillation

   (iv) Patients who survive cardiac arrest and are symptomatic despite therapy should be considered for AICD

(f) Direct-current cardioversion may be necessary for tachyarrhythmias resistant to pharmacologic therapy and/or those that are producing hemodynamic instability; it can be used at all stages of pregnancy without significant fetal complications

Anemia

1. Dilutional anemia of pregnancy
   (a) Plasma volume increases by ~50% and red blood cell (RBC) mass increases by ~30%
   (b) Average Hgb at term gestation is 11.6 g/dL
   (c) If Hgb is <10.5 g/dL, the cause is something other than dilutional anemia
   (d) Hgb ≥ 14.5 g/dL may reflect inadequate volume expansion
2. Thalassemia
   (a) Microcytic, hemolytic anemia due to a reduced synthesis of one of the polypeptide globin chains
   (b) Leads to: imbalance in globin chain synthesis; defective hemoglobin synthesis; and erythrocyte damage resulting from excess globin subunits
   (c) Alpha-thalassemia – decreased alpha-chain production. Four types because there are four alpha chain genes:
       (i) Silent carrier (three functioning genes) – seen in 30% of African Americans
       (ii) α-thalassemia trait (two functioning genes) – 3% of African Americans. Consider in black women with microcytic anemia that does not respond to iron therapy
       (iii) Hemoglobin H disease (one functioning gene) – moderately severe anemia, splenomegaly, fatigue, and generalized discomfort
       (iv) α^0-thalassemia or Bart's hydrops (no functioning genes) – beta chains form tetramers without alpha chains. Generally incompatible with life. Individuals die *in utero* or shortly after birth of hydrops fetalis
   (d) Beta-thalassemia – decreased beta-chain production. Two genes for beta chains, thus types of thalassemia:
       (i) B^0-thalassemia (AKA β-thalassemia major or Cooley's anemia) – no beta chain formation
           1. Severe anemia develops in the first few months of extra-uterine life
           2. Expansion of marrow cavities due to increased erythropoietin production causes skeletal abnormalities and pathologic fractures

© Springer Nature Switzerland AG 2019
C. Wasson et al., *Absolute Obstetric Anesthesia Review*,
https://doi.org/10.1007/978-3-319-96980-0_38

3. Splenomegaly leads to leukopenia and thrombocytopenia
4. Transfusions are required to maintain life, leading to iron accumulation, which may lead to DM, adrenal insufficiency, infertility, and heart failure
5. Treatment: transfusion to maintain Hgb > 10 g/dL, splenectomy, and iron chelation therapy
   (a) Normal Hgb 2 g/dL at age <2
   (b) Typical Hgb 4–10 g/dL age 2–12
6. Rare for these patients to conceive. If they do, higher incidence of spontaneous abortion, intrauterine fetal demise (IUFD), and IUGR

(ii) β^+-thalassemia (AKA β-thalassemia minor) – some beta-chain production exists. Mild anemia (Hgb 9–11) and benign clinical course.
   1. Tolerate pregnancy well
(iii) Excess α chains precipitate and form inclusion bodies in RBC precursors

3. Sickle cell disease – RBC undergo sickling when they are deoxygenated, causing clinical signs/symptoms
   (a) Homozygous for abnormal Hgb (hemoglobin SS or sickle cell anemia)
      (i) Valine is substituted for glutamic acid as the sixth amino acid in the beta chains
      (ii) Oxygen tension is the most important determinant of sickling; Hgb S begins to aggregate at a P_{O2} of less than 50 mmHg
      (iii) Other factors that increase sickling:
         1. Hgb S concentration >50% of the total Hgb
         2. Dehydration (due to increased blood viscosity)
         3. Hypotension, which causes vascular stasis
         4. Hypothermia
         5. Acidosis
      (iv) Sickled cells can form aggregates and cause vaso-occlusive disease, which may lead to infarctive crises (most often occurring in chest, abdomen, back, and long bones), CVA, and, rarely, peripheral neuropathy
      (v) Increased risk of pneumonia and pyelonephritis in pregnant patients with sickle cell disease than in other pregnant patients
      (vi) Pregnancy exacerbates complications of sickle cell anemia
         1. Pulmonary embolism (PE) and infection are the leading cause of death
         2. Fetal mortality is elevated (~20%)
         3. Increased incidence of preterm labor, placental abruption, placenta previa, and hypertensive disorders of pregnancy
      (vii) Principles of anesthetic management:
         1. Use crystalloid to maintain intravascular volume
         2. Transfuse RBCs to maintain O_2-carrying capacity
         3. Supplemental O_2 and use pulse oximetry

       4. Maintain normothermia

       5. Prevent peripheral venous stasis

(b) Heterozygous for abnormal Hgb (hemoglobin SA or sickle cell trait)

   (i) Pregnant women with sickle cell trait are at increased risk for asymptomatic bacteriuria, pyelonephritis, and preeclampsia

(c) Double heterozygous for abnormal Hgb (hemoglobin SC or sickle cell hemoglobin C disease)

   (i) Hgb SC disease have increased tendency to develop marrow necrosis, which predisposes to fat emboli

4. Autoimmune hemolytic anemia

(a) Four main types:

   (i) Incomplete warm autoantibodies

      1. Usually IgG

      2. RBC destruction in the spleen

      3. Treatment: corticosteroids, splenectomy, gamma-globulin

  (ii) Complete warm autoantibodies (type I and II)

      1. IgM antibodies

      2. RBC destruction in the liver or intracellular

      3. Treatment: corticosteroids, splenectomy, plasma exchange, corticosteroids

  (iii) Cold autoagglutinins and hemolysis

      1. IgM antibodies

      2. RBC destruction intracellular

      3. Treatment: corticosteroids and keeping the patient warm

  (iv) Biphasic hemolysins (acute and chronic)

      1. IgG antibodies

      2. RBC destruction intracellular

      3. Treatment: treat underlying infection, plasmapheresis, chlorambucil

(b) Etiologies:

   (i) Primary or idiopathic

  (ii) Secondary

      1. Neoplasms

      2. Drug-related

      3. Infections

      4. Connective tissue diseases

      5. Other diseases

      6. Pregnancy

Thrombocytopenic Coagulopathies

39

1. Autoimmune thrombocytopenic purpura (AKA idiopathic thrombocytopenic purpura (ITP))
   (a) IgG initiated platelet destruction
   (b) Consider when platelet count is <100,000/mm³ with normal or higher numbers of megakaryocytes
   (c) Differential includes nonimmunologic (gestational or essential thrombocytopenia, preeclampsia, DIC, or TTP) and immunologic (drug-induced thrombocytopenia, post-transfusion purpura, and pseudothrombocytopenia)
      (i) Pseudothrombocytopenia is a lab artifact due to chelation of Ca^{++} by EDTA and platelet clumping
   (d) Administer corticosteroids if platelet count is <20,000/mm³ prior to onset of labor or <50,000/mm³ at the time of delivery
   (e) IVIG is administered if there is no response to corticosteroids
2. Thrombotic thrombocytopenic purpura (TTP)
   (a) Defined by classic pentad: fever, thrombocytopenia, microangiopathic hemolytic anemia, neurologic signs (e.g., photophobia, headache, seizures), and renal failure
   (b) Treatment: infusion of plasma with plasmapheresis, IVIG, prednisone, and infusion of prostacyclin
   (c) Avoid platelet transfusion
   (d) Neuraxial anesthesia is not recommended due to presence of coagulopathy
3. Drug-induced platelet disorders
   (a) Drugs can accelerate platelet destruction, but these drugs are not often used in OB patients (e.g., quinidine, quinine, gold salts, heparin)
   (b) Drugs may also decrease platelet function (e.g., aspirin)
      (i) Aspirin and nonsteroidal anti-inflammatory drugs inhibit cyclooxygenase
      (ii) Prostaglandin E_1 and prostacyclin stimulate adenyl cyclase

© Springer Nature Switzerland AG 2019
C. Wasson et al., *Absolute Obstetric Anesthesia Review*,
https://doi.org/10.1007/978-3-319-96980-0_39

        (iii) Caffeine and theophylline inhibit phosphodiesterase

        (iv) Penicillin, cephalosporins, hydroxyethyl starch, dextran, and heparin also affect platelets

    (c) Recent ingestion of aspirin or other NSAIDs do not contraindicate that administration of neuraxial anesthesia

Other Hematologic Disorders

40

1. von Willebrand's disease – autosomal dominant
   (a) von Willebrand's factor is synthesized by endothelial cells and megakaryocytes. Production of vWF is increased in normal pregnancy, so antenatal bleeding is rare in women with type I disease
   (b) Two primary roles in coagulation:
      (i) forms a complex with factor VIII, which decreases the excretion of factor VIII. Factor VIII degrades rapidly when not bound to vWF (half-life of Factor VIII increases to 8–12 hours when bound to vWF compared to 1–2 hours in the absence of vWF)
         1. Thus, factor VIII may be decreased in von Willebrand's disease
      (ii) mediates platelet adhesion by binding to platelets and collagen
   (c) Platelet function is affected and bleeding time is prolonged in von Willebrand's disease
   (d) Several subtypes exist. Treat type I or IIa with DDAVP
      (i) FFP or cryoprecipitate is administered to those without response to DDAVP
2. Other coagulation factor deficiencies
   (a) Hemophilia A (factor VIII deficiency) – X-linked recessive
   (b) Hemophilia B (factor IX deficiency) – X-linked recessive
3. Disseminated intravascular coagulation (DIC)
   (a) Abnormal activation of the coagulation system, causing:
      (i) Formation of large amounts of thrombin
      (ii) Depletion of coagulation factors
      (iii) Activation of the fibrinolytic system
      (iv) Hemorrhage
   (b) Most common causes in OB population: preeclampsia, placental abruption, sepsis, retained dead fetus syndrome, and amniotic fluid embolism

© Springer Nature Switzerland AG 2019

C. Wasson et al., *Absolute Obstetric Anesthesia Review*,

https://doi.org/10.1007/978-3-319-96980-0_40

(c) Lab findings: thrombocytopenia; decreased fibrinogen and antithrombin III concentrations; variable increases in PT, aPTT, thrombin, and reptilase times; and higher concentrations of D-dimer, fibrin monomer, and fibrin degradation products

(d) Treatment: treat or remove precipitating cause

4. Hypercoagulable states

(a) Increased risk of venous thrombosis with surgery, pregnancy, oral contraceptive use, and immobilization

(b) Patients with hypercoagulation have increased incidence of IUGR, preeclampsia, placental abruption, and IUFD

(c) Protein C deficiency

(i) Levels normally increase ~35% during pregnancy

(ii) Produced in the liver and needs vitamin K for synthesis

(iii) Inhibits activated factor V and VIII

(d) Factor V Leiden

(i) Mutant factor V Leiden protein persists longer in the circulation leading to hypercoagulable state

(e) Protein S deficiency

(i) Levels normally decrease during pregnancy

(ii) Produced in the liver and depends on vit K for synthesis

(f) Antithrombin III deficiency

(i) Synthesized in the liver and endothelial cells

(ii) Inactivates thrombin and factors IXa, Xa, Xia, and XIIa. Heparin acts by potentiating the activity of antithrombin III. Heparin may not work if antithrombin III levels are deficient.

(iii) Quantitative and qualitative deficiencies both exist

(g) Lupus anticoagulant – patients are hypercoagulable

Hypertension (HTN)

41

1. Result in fetal complications (e.g., preterm birth, IUGR, and fetal/neonatal death)
2. Chronic HTN
   (a) Pre-pregnancy HTN or HTN that fails to resolve after delivery
   (b) Chronic HTN with superimposed preeclampsia is when preeclampsia develops in a woman who had chronic HTN before pregnancy
3. Gestational HTN – most common cause of HTN during pregnancy
   (a) Elevated BP after 20 weeks' gestation that resolves by 12 weeks postpartum
4. Preeclampsia
   (a) New onset of HTN (BP > 140/90 mmHg, on two occasions at least 4 hours apart) and proteinuria after 20 weeks' gestation
   (b) Consider diagnosis in absence of proteinuria if patient has:
      (i) Persistent epigastric or RUQ pain
      (ii) Persistent cerebral symptoms
      (iii) Fetal growth restriction
      (iv) Thrombocytopenia, or
      (v) Elevated serum liver enzymes to twice normal concentration, or serum Cr > 1.1 mg/dL, or doubling of serum Cr concentration in the absence of other renal disease
   (c) HELLP syndrome: hemolysis, elevated liver enzymes, and low platelets in a woman with preeclampsia
   (d) Partner-related risk factors for developing preeclampsia: limited maternal exposure to paternal sperm antigens prior to conception (e.g., mulliparity, teenagers, parous women conceiving with a new partner, using barrier methods prior to conception, conceiving with donated sperm)
   (e) Non-partner-related risk factors: history of preeclampsia in a prior pregnancy; advanced maternal age (>35); family history of preeclampsia; history of prior placental abruption, IUGR, or fetal death; non-hispanic black race; history of chronic HTN, obesity, DM, or thrombotic vascular disease

© Springer Nature Switzerland AG 2019
C. Wasson et al., *Absolute Obstetric Anesthesia Review*,
https://doi.org/10.1007/978-3-319-96980-0_41

(f) Affects multiple organ systems:
  (i) Neurologic: severe headache, visual disturbances, hyperexcitability, hyperreflexia, and coma. Intracranial hemorrage is the most common cause of death in preeclampsia. Highly associated with SBP > 160 mmHg
  (ii) Airway: exaggerated upper airway narrowing due to pharyngolaryngeal edema
  (iii) Pulmonary edema due to decreased plasma albumin concentration
  (iv) Cardiovascular: increased vascular tone and greater sensitivity to vasoconstrictor influences
  (v) Hematologic: thrombocytopenia and DIC
    1. Mild preeclampsia is hypercoagulable
    2. Severe preeclampsia is hypocoagulable
  (vi) Hepatic: periportal hemorrhage and fibrin deposition in hepatic sinusoids, rarely leading to hepatic rupture
  (vii) Renal: persistent proteinuria, changes in GFR, and hyperuricemia
(g) Delivery is the only cure
(h) Treatment
  (i) Hydralazine – treatment of choice for severe HTN in preeclampsia
  (ii) Labetalol – alpha- and beta-adrenergic receptor antagonist with a 1:7 ratio of alpha- to beta-antagonism
    1. Avoid in patients with severe asthma or CHF
  (iii) Esmolol – can cross placenta and cause fetal bradycardia
  (iv) Sodium nitroprusside – used for refractory preeclampsia.
    1. Causes release of nitric oxide, which relaxes arterial vessels and reduces both afterload and venous return.
    2. Sodium nitroprusside is metabolized to cyanide, which undergoes placental transfer, causing risk of fetal cyanide toxicity
  (v) Nifedipine – relaxes arterial and arteriolar smooth muscle. It interacts with magnesium sulfate causing severe hypotension and neuromuscular blockade
(i) Seizure prophylaxis with magnesium sulfate in women with severe preeclampsia is routine
  (i) Side effects of magnesium: chest pain and tightness, palpitations, nausea, blurred vision, sedation, transient hypotension, and rarely pulmonary edema
  (ii) Therapeutic range is 5–9 mg/dL
    1. Patellar reflexes are lost at 12 mg/dL
    2. Respiratory arrest occurs at 15–20 mg/dL
    3. Asystole occurs at >25 mg/dL
  (iii) Treatment of magnesium toxicity: stop infusion and give IV calcium gluconate (1 g) over 10 min
(j) Severe preeclampsia has an increased risk of morbidity and mortality, including HELLP syndrome, CVA, pulmonary edema, renal failure, placental abruption, and eclampsia

(k) Platelet count can fall precipitously in HELLP syndrome and should be re-evaluated prior to administration of neuraxial anesthesia

    (i) Platelets <50,000/mm^3 are at significantly higher risk of bleeding, necessitating GA for cesarean

(l) Four considerations when administering neuraxial anesthesia to preeclamptic patients

    (i) Assessment of coagulation status

        1. Platelet >100,000/mm^3 has rare coagulopathy

        2. <100,000/mm^3 may need PT/PTT prior to neuraxial to check coagulation

        3. Trend in platelet count is more important than a set number in preeclamptic patients

        4. In normal pregnancy (without preeclampsia), platelet >75,000/mm^3 appears adequate for neuraxial anesthesia

        5. Platelet count <50,000/mm^3 precludes neuraxial administration

        6. Check platelet count again prior to removal of epidural catheter

    (ii) IV hydration prior to epidural administration of local anesthetic

        1. Careful IV fluid infusion due to increased risk of pulmonary edema in preeclampsia

    (iii) Treatment of hypotension

        1. Use smaller doses of ephedrine (2.5 mg) or phenylephrine (25–50 μg) to effect since preeclamptic patients are more sensitive to vasopressors

    (iv) Use of an epi-containing local anesthetic solution

        1. Hypothetical risk of causing hypertensive crisis in preeclamptic women, but no randomized controlled trials have shown increased risk

        2. Patients on beta-blockers (e.g., labetalol) do not have tachycardic response to epinephrine

5. Eclampsia

  (a) New onset seizures in a woman with preeclampsia

  (b) Anesthetic management is same as that of severe preeclampsia

  (c) During immediate delivery in a woman with ongoing seizures, induction with propofol or pentothal will terminate the seizure.

    (i) Employ hyperventilation with caution due to reduction in cerebral blood flow without decrease in metabolic rate

    (ii) Avoid hypoventilation, as can lead to hypercarbia, which lowers seizure threshold

    (iii) Avoid hypoxia, hyperthermia, and hyperglycemia as these can exacerbate neurologic injury

Neurologic Disorders

1. Multiple sclerosis
   (a) Two general patterns of presentation:
      (i) Exacerbating remitting: attacks appear abruptly and resolve over several months
      (ii) Chronic progressive: deficits become more progressive and debilitating over time
   (b) Pathologic findings: inflammation and loss of myelin in the CNS
   (c) Relapse rate is slightly decreased during pregnancy, but increases during the first 3–6 months postpartum
      (i) Likely due to stress, exhaustion, infection, loss of antenatal immunosuppression, and postpartum decline in concentrations of reproductive hormones
   (d) Neuraxial anesthesia is the preferred anesthetic technique used for cesarean delivery.
   (e) For labor analgesia with epidural, use a diluted solution of local anesthetic when possible.
   (f) The type of anesthesia selected for cesarean section does not appear to influence the relapse rate
2. Spinal cord injury
   (a) Cord injury below S2 experience pain during labor
      (i) Lesion above T10 do NOT experience labor pain
   (b) Autonomic hyperreflexia occurs with injuries at or above T6
      (i) Life-threatening complication from absence of central inhibition on the sympathetic neurons below the injury
      (ii) Noxious stimuli, bladder or bowel distention, and uterine contractions send afferent impulses by the dorsal spinal root, which synapse with sympathetic neurons and cause impulse to propagate both cephalad and caudad in the sympathetic chain. There is no central inhibition, so

sympathetic hyperactivity occurs, causing severe systemic hypertension secondary to vasoconstriction below the level of the lesion. In response to this systemic hypertension, the baroreceptors of the aortic and carotid bodies cause bradycardia and vasodilation above the level of the lesion.

    (iii) Distinguished from other causes of intrapartum hypertension by cyclical HTN (i.e., BP increases during contractions and decreases between contractions)

    (iv) Best way to prevent/treat is with neuraxial anesthesia

(c) Pregnancy may aggravate medical complications of spinal cord injury:

    (i) Pulmonary: decreased respiratory reserve, atelectasis, pneumonia, impaired cough

    (ii) Hematologic: anemia, deep venous thrombosis (DVT), thrombotic phenomena

    (iii) Urogenital: chronic urinary tract infection (UTI), urinary tract calculi, proteinuria, renal insufficiency

    (iv) Dermatologic: decubitus ulcers

    (v) Cardiovascular: HTN, autonomic hyperreflexia

3. Myasthenia gravis

(a) Autoimmune disorder with muscle weakness that worsens with activity

    (i) Antibodies against the nicotinic acetylcholine receptor on the neuromuscular end plate of skeletal muscle (smooth muscle and cardiac muscle are NOT affected)

(b) Two types of crises:

    (i) Cholinergic crisis: due to excess muscarinic effects of anticholinesterase mediations

       1. Symptoms: muscle weakness, respiratory difficulty or failure, increased sweating, salivation, bronchial secretions, and miosis

    (ii) Myasthenic crisis: due to worsening of the disease

       1. Symptoms: severe muscle weakness, including greater weakness of respiratory muscles

    (iii) Distinguish between the two by administering edrophonium

       1. If symptoms improve, it's a myasthenic crisis and needs a higher dose of anticholinesterase medications

       2. If symptoms do not improve, it's a cholinergic crisis

(c) 1/3 of patients' symptoms worsen during pregnancy; 1/3 improve; 1/3 stay unchanged

(d) Caution with use of opioids due to respiratory depression and worsening respiratory compromise

(e) Neuraxial anesthesia is preferred for labor analgesia

    (i) Ester local anesthetics may have prolonged effect because plasma cholinesterase activity is decreased in patients taking anticholinesterase drugs

    (ii) Amides should be used to decrease the risk of local anesthetic toxicity

(f) Risk for postoperative ventilation:
  (i) Duration of myasthenia greater than 6 years
  (ii) History of chronic respiratory disease
  (iii) Pyridostigmine dose higher than 750 mg/day
  (iv) Vital capacity less than 2.9 L
  (v) Female gender
  (vi) $FEF_{25-75\%}$ less than 3.3 L/s and less than 85% predicted
  (vii) FVC less than 2.6 L/s and less than 78% predicted
  (viii) $MEF_{50\%}$ less than 3.9 L/s and less than 80% predicted
(g) Effects on anesthetic management
  (i) Patients are extremely sensitive to non-depolarizing muscle relaxants, and resistant to depolarizing muscle relaxants (e.g. succinylcholine)
  (ii) Avoid magnesium sulfate, aminoglycosides, fluoroquinolones, tetracyclines, and macrolides antibiotics.
  (iii) Levetiracetam is safe to use as seizure prophylaxis for pre-eclamptic patients.
4. Epilepsy: recurrent seizure activity in the absence of metabolic disorders or acute brain disease
  (a) Two major types: partial and generalized
  (b) 1/3 of patients will have increased seizure frequency during pregnancy; ½ will have no change
  (c) Hypoxia and acidosis that occur during generalized seizures may lead to fetal compromise or intrauterine fetal death
  (d) Epileptic women are 2× as likely to have preeclampsia, preterm labor, and placental abnormalities
  (e) Infants of epileptic women are 2× as likely to have adverse outcomes (i.e., IUFD, cesarean delivery, neonatal and perinatal death, low birth weight, and abnormal development)
    (i) Most common malformations are cleft lip and palate, and cardiac, neural tube, and urogenital defects
  (f) Infants of mothers undergoing long-term antiepileptic therapy are at risk for deficiency of vitamin K-dependent clotting factors (due to liver enzyme induction)
  (g) Some antiepileptic medications induce liver enzymes, which may lead to rapid breakdown of anesthetic agents that are metabolized by the liver
  (h) No contraindication to administration of neuraxial analgesia or anesthesia
  (i) If GA is necessary, avoid ketamine, enflurane, and meperidine, as these may lower the seizure threshold
5. Myotonia and myotonic dystrophy
  (a) Myotonia: prolonged contraction of certain muscles after stimulation, followed by delayed relaxation
  (b) Myotonic dystrophies are genetically and phenotypically heterogenous group of neuromuscular disorders characterized by skeletal muscle weakness and myotonia, cardiac conduction abnormalities, cataracts, hypogammaglobulinemia, and insulin resistance

    (c) Muscle weakness may prolong the second stage of labor

    (d) Poor uterine contractions may result in prolonged labor, uterine atony, and increased risk of postpartum hemorrhage

    (e) Neuraxial anesthesia is preferred due to higher risk of apnea with opioids in these patients

6. Muscular dystrophy

    (a) Progressive degeneration of skeletal muscle with intact innervation

    (b) Duchenne and Becker muscular dystrophies are X-linked recessive disorders and occur almost exclusively in males

    (c) Neuraxial anesthesia is preferred

7. Neurocutaneous syndromes (AKA phakomatoses)

    (a) Neurofibromatosis (NF) (type 1 and 2)

        (i) Excess proliferation of neural crest elements (e.g., Schwann cells, melanocytes, and fibroblasts)

        (ii) Clinical manifestations: hyperpigmented lesions (café-au-lait spots) with cutaneous and subcutaneous tumors

        (iii) Severe kyphoscoliosis may be present and complicate the administration of neuraxial anesthesia

        (iv) Lesions can involve the neck and larynx, and are common in patients with NF1.

        (v) Asymptomatic paraspinal and intracranial tumors may be present; careful clinical and radiologic evaluations may be indicated prior to neuraxial anesthesia

    (b) Tuberous sclerosis

        (i) Characterized by epilepsy, mental retardation, and adenoma sebaceum

        (ii) Few reports of pregnancy in women with tuberous sclerosis

    (c) Angiomatoses with CNS abnormalities (e.g., Sturge-Weber syndrome, Klippel-Trenaunay-Weber syndrome, epidermal nevus syndrome, Osler-Rendu-Weber disease, von Hippel-Lindau disease, Louis-Bar disease, and Fabry disease)

        (i) Few reports of pregnancy in women with these disorders

8. Landry-Guillain-Barre syndrome (AKA acute idiopathic polyneuritis)

    (a) Inflammatory demyelinating illness

    (b) Weakness first of the limbs, followed by the trunk, neck, and facial muscles

        (i) Loss of reflexes, total motor paralysis, and respiratory failure can occur

        (ii) Sensory loss typically does not occur

    (c) Treatment is supportive, including mechanical ventilation

    (d) Epidurals have been used successfully in parturients with Guillain-Barre

    (e) Avoid succinylcholine if GA is necessary

9. Polio

    (a) Affects motor neurons in the cerebral cortex, brainstem, and spinal cord

    (b) Asymmetric flaccid paralysis develops over several days

    (c) Epidurals have been used successfully

10. Brain neoplasms
    (a) Gliomas are the most common intracranial neoplasm
    (b) Increased risk of herniation during painful uterine contractions
    (c) Epidurals are controversial
        (i) They prevent the increase in intracranial pressure (ICP) during the second stage of labor, but unintentional dural puncture can result in herniation
    (d) GA is preferred for cesarean deliveries in patients with brain neoplasms
11. Idiopathic Intracranial HTN (AKA pseudotumor cerebri)
    (a) Increase in ICP with normal CSF composition, in the absence of hydrocephalus or a mass lesion
    (b) Herniation does not occur with lumbar puncture due to global increase in ICP, so spinal anesthesia is safe
12. Maternal hydrocephalus with shunt   .
    (a) Most common causes of hydrocephalus: intracranial hemorrhage in preterm infants, fetal and neonatal infections, Arnold-Chiari malformation, aqueductal stenosis, and the Dandy-Walker syndrome
    (b) Ventriculoatrial or ventriculoperitoneal shunts are placed for treatment
    (c) Epidural and intrathecal anesthesia have both been used successfully in these patients
13. Intracerebral hemorrhage
    (a) Most commonly due to AV malformation or aneurysm
    (b) Neuraxial analgesia is preferred during labor to prevent hemodynamic instability and aneurysm or AV malformation rupture
14. Cerebral vein thrombosis
    (a) Obstetric delivery may be a precipitating factor for sinus thrombosis in a person with a genetically increased risk
    (b) Patients are treated with anticoagulation, so neuraxial anesthesia is contraindicated
    (c) Avoid systemic hypotension during GA, as this may decreases cerebral perfusion pressure and blood flow to injured areas
15. Motor neuron disorders
    (a) Progressive muscular weakness and atrophy, alone or in conjunction with sensory deficits
    (b) Examples include amyotrophic lateral sclerosis, spinal muscular atrophy, and peroneal muscular atrophy (AKA Charcot-Marie-Tooth disease)
    (c) Assessment of pulmonary function is important
    (d) Neuraxial anesthesia has been successfully used
16. Isolated mononeuropathies during pregnancy
    (a) Bell's palsy: acute onset facial nerve paralysis. No contraindication to neuraxial analgesia
    (b) Carpal tunnel syndrome: common during pregnancy. Compression of the median nerve in the flexor retinaculum.
    (c) Meralgia paresthetica: sensory loss and paresthesias in the lateral thigh due to compression of the lateral femoral cutaneous nerve

Asthma

43

1. Three characteristic findings: reversible airway obstruction, airway inflammation, and airway hyperresponsiveness
2. The underlying cause of symptoms is unknown
3. Asthma may subjectively improve, worsen, or stay the same during pregnancy
4. Asthma exacerbations occur during labor and delivery and are more frequent after cesarean than vaginal delivery (41% vs 4%)
5. Increased incidence of preeclampsia, cesarean delivery, low-birth-weight infants, preterm labor, antepartum and postpartum hemorrhage, and perinatal mortality
6. Asthma medications are generally safe for the fetus
   (a) Bronchodilators
       (i) Beta-adrenergic agonists cause direct airway smooth muscle relaxation, enhance mucociliary transport, decrease airway edema, and inhibit cholinergic neurotransmission
       (ii) Methylxanthines (e.g., theophylline) inhibit intracellular phosphodiesterase and increase concentrations of cAMP
       (iii) Anticholinergic agents (e.g., ipratropium) block muscarinic receptors on airway smooth muscle to cause bronchodilation
       (iv) Magnesium sulfate antagonizes calcium, leading to airway smooth muscle relaxation. Use is limited to acute bronchospasm
   (b) Anti-inflammatory agents (e.g., corticosteroids, cromolyn, leukotriene receptor antagonists, and leukotriene synthesis inhibitors)
       (i) Corticosteroids decrease cellular infiltration and mediator release, reduce airway permeability, and up-regulate beta-adrenergic system
       (ii) Inhaled corticosteroids are not associated with increased perinatal risk
           1. Need careful glucose monitoring, especially in women also receiving beta-adrenergic agonists
           2. Moderate doses of inhaled corticosteroids do not produce adrenocortical suppression, so steroid stress dose is not needed

© Springer Nature Switzerland AG 2019
C. Wasson et al., *Absolute Obstetric Anesthesia Review*,
https://doi.org/10.1007/978-3-319-96980-0_43

    (iii) Cromolyn sodium reduces inflammation by stabilizing mast cells and is safe in pregnancy

    (iv) Leukotriene receptor antagonists and leukotriene synthesis inhibitors are not well studied in pregnancy

7. Relative contraindication to carboprost/hemabate for the treatment of postpartum hemorrhage

8. Analgesic regimens for asthmatics include systemic opioids, paracervical block, pudendal nerve block, lumbar sympathetic block, and epidural or spinal analgesia with local anesthetics, opioids, or both

    (a) High dose systemic opioids should be avoided due to risk of respiratory depression

    (b) Paracervical and pudendal nerve blocks provide analgesia without sedation or paralysis of the respiratory muscles. These are performed by the obstetrician

    (c) An epidural has a risk of high thoracic motor block and respiratory insufficiency. Maintain sensory level at T10 to minimize this risk.

    (d) Epidural provides the advantage of avoiding the risks of general endotracheal anesthesia for an urgent/emergent cesarean

9. Neuraxial is preferred to GA for cesarean as it has a lower incidence of bronchospasm than GA in asthmatic patients

    (a) Neuraxial anesthesia may be hazardous in an unstable asthmatic who requires accessory muscles of respiration because of the impaired ventilator capacity with a high thoracic motor block

    (b) Ketamine relaxes airway smooth muscle and is a good induction agent for asthmatic subjects

    (c) Pretreatment with beta-adrenergic agonist can attenuate reflex-induced bronchoconstriction after intubation

    (d) IV lidocaine inhibits airway reflexes and helps attenuate irritant-induced bronchoconstriction

    (e) Bronchodilators may be used if bronchospasm occurs, but the most effective bronchodilators (i.e., beta-adrenergic agonists) also relax the uterus and may lead to uterine atony. This effect is minimized by administering it via aerosol.

Other Respiratory Disorders

44

1. Cigarette smoking
   (a) Significant, preventable cause of maternal morbidity and prenatal mortality
   (b) Causes alterations in small airway function, increased mucus secretion, and impaired ciliary transport
   (c) Marked increase in postop pulmonary complications
   (d) Associated with IUGR, preterm birth, and perinatal mortality
   (e) Anesthetic management of partiurient smokers is the same as that for asthmatic partiurients
2. Cystic fibrosis
   (a) Lethal, autosomal recessive disorder
   (b) Due to a defect in the cAMP-mediated activation of the Cl⁻ conductance in the epithelium
   (c) Spontaneous pneumothorax is common
   (d) Chronic airway obstruction and impaired mucus clearance increases the frequency of pulmonary infection, often with *P. aeruginosa*
   (e) Chronic hypoxemia and lung disease may cause pulmonary HTN and cor pulmonale
   (f) Pregnancy may have negative effects on the clinical course of cystic fibrosis, but it does not appear to affect long-term survival
   (g) Higher risk of low birth weight infants and preterm delivery
   (h) Anesthetic goals for pain relief during labor include avoiding high thoracic motor block and respiratory depression
      (i) Parenteral opioids may worsen pulmonary function
   (i) For cesarean delivery, there is no difference in outcome between GA and neuraxial
      (i) Neuraxial avoids ETT (which may become obstructed with secretions) and positive-pressure ventilation (which may enlarge a preexisting pneumothorax)

© Springer Nature Switzerland AG 2019
C. Wasson et al., *Absolute Obstetric Anesthesia Review*,
https://doi.org/10.1007/978-3-319-96980-0_44

           1. May require frequent suctioning of ETT

           2. Avoid NO_2 due to risk of pneumothorax

     (ii) Neuraxial has the risk of a high thoracic motor block

3. Respiratory failure

   (a) Mortality from respiratory failure during pregnancy is high

   (b) Most significant effect on pregnancy is the decreased delivery of oxygen to the fetus due to maternal hypotension or hypoxemia

   (c) Many causes during pregnancy:

     (i) ARDS due to:

       1. Infection (bacterial or viral pneumonia, endometritis, pyelonephritis, sepsis, preeclampsia)

       2. Hemorrhage (multiple transfusions or DIC)

       3. Aspiration of gastric contents

       4. Embolism

       5. Drugs (salicylates or opioids)

     (ii) PE from thromboembolism, amniotic fluid embolism (AFE), or venous air embolism (VAE)

     (iii) Cystic fibrosis

     (iv) Pulmonary edema due to beta-adrenergic receptor agonists (e.g., ritodrine or terbutaline) or cardiogenic

   (d) Treatment is the same as for nonpregnant patients

   (e) Analgesia for labor of mechanically ventilated patients can be achieved with IV opioids, which is often used for sedation

     (i) General anesthesia is convenient for cesarean

   (f) For patients not mechanically ventilated, epidural analgesia helps reduce O_2 consumption, which may be beneficial. Assess the underlying condition, including intravascular volume, coagulation status, and presence or absence of infection

Renal Disorders

45

1. Renal parenchymal disease
   (a) Glomerulopathies
      (i) Nephritic syndromes: inflammatory or necrotizing lesions
      (ii) Nephrotic syndromes: abnormal permeability to protein and other macromolecules
   (b) Tubulointerstitial disease: abnormal tubular function (i.e., interstitial nephritis, renal cystic disease, renal neoplasia, and functional tubular defects)
   (c) Pregnancy does not alter the natural course of renal disease in women with mild antenatal renal insufficiency, but it often causes deterioration of renal function in parturients with moderate or severe antenatal renal insufficiency
   (d) Obstetric complications from chronic renal disease include IUGR, preterm delivery, HTN, preeclampsia, an increased cesarean delivery rate, and higher risk of neonatal mortality
   (e) Recombinant human erythropoietin improves maternal anemia during pregnancy
   (f) Abnormalities that may affect anesthetic management in chronic renal failure:
      (i) Cardiovascular: HTN, fluid overload, ventricular hypertrophy, accelerated atherosclerosis, uremic pericarditis, and uremic cardiomyopathy
      (ii) Gastrointestinal: delayed gastric emptying, increased gastric acidity, hepatic venous congestion, hepatitis (viral or drug-induced), malnutrition
      1. Chronic uremia causes delayed gastric emptying and hyperacidity
      (iii) Pulmonary: increased risk of difficult airway and recurrent pulmonary infections
      1. Increased risk of aspiration pneumonitis due to delayed gastric emptying and hyperacidity

© Springer Nature Switzerland AG 2019
C. Wasson et al., *Absolute Obstetric Anesthesia Review*,
https://doi.org/10.1007/978-3-319-96980-0_45

(iv) Metabolic and endocrine: hyperkalemia, metabolic acidosis, hyponatremia, hypocalcemia, hypermagnesemia, hypoglycemia, decreased
protein binding of drugs

(v) Hematologic: anemia, platelet dysfunction, decreased coagulation factors, leukocyte dysfunction

1. Uremia causes functional platelet defects and a prolonged bleeding
time that dialysis reverses

(vi) Neurologic: autonomic neuropathy, mental status changes, peripheral
neuropathy, restless leg syndrome, seizure disorder

(g) Hypovolemia and autonomic neuropathy may cause profound hypotension
during sympathetic blockade. Minimize the risk with prehydration and slow
induction of epidural

2. Acute renal failure (ARF)

(a) Defined by a sharp increase in plasma creatinine (>0.8 mg/dL) and BUN
(>13 mg/dL) concentrations.

(b) Subdivided by etiology (i.e., prerenal, postrenal, intrarenal)

(i) Prerenal urinary indices show $U_{osm} > 500$ mOsm/kg H_2O,
$U_{Na} < 20$ mEq/L, FENA < 1%, and a urinary-to-plasma creatinine ratio
>40

1. Due to hyperemesis gravidarum, uterine hemorrhage, or heart
failure

(ii) Intrarenal urinary indices show $U_{osm} < 350$ mOsm/kg H_2O,
$U_{Na} > 40$ mEq/L, FENA > 1%, and a urinary-to-plasma creatinine ratio
<20

1. Due to acute tubular necrosis (ATN), septic abortion, AFE, drug-
induced acute interstitial nephritis, acute glomerulonephritis, bilateral renal cortical necrosis, acute pyelonephritis, preeclampsia/
eclampsia, HELLP syndrome, acute fatty liver of pregnancy, and
idiopathic postpartum renal failure

(iii) Postrenal due to urolithiasis or ureteral obstruction by the gravid uterus

(c) Leading cause of pregnancy-related ARF in developing countries is septic
abortion

(d) Most common cause in developed countries is severe preeclampsia/eclamp-
sia, acute pyelonephritis of pregnancy, and bilateral renal cortical necrosis

(e) ATN is due to nephrotoxic drugs, AFE, rhabdomyolysis, IUFD, and prolonged renal ischemia from hemorrhagic or septic shock

(i) UA shows brown epithelial cell casts and coarse granular casts

(f) Acute interstitial nephritis is caused by NSAIDs and some antibiotics.
Eosinophilia and urine eosinophils are seen

(g) Bilateral renal cortical necrosis is most commonly caused by placental
abruption. Pathogenesis is unclear.

(h) Neuraxial anesthesia may be administered in the absence of coagulopathy,
thrombocytopenia, and hypovolemia

(i) Epidural may be preferred over spinal when intravascular volume status
is questionable

3. Renal transplantation
   (a) Increased pregnancy complications: IUGR, IUFD, preterm delivery, spontaneous abortion, and HTN
   (b) Pregnancy does not affect long-term outcome of renal allograft
   (c) Fetus will be exposed to immunosuppressant drugs and may be adversely affected
   (d) Stress-dose corticosteroid is indicated in cesarean deliveries
   (e) No contraindications to neuraxial anesthesia, but strict aseptic technique must be maintained
4. Urolithiasis
   (a) Most stones are calcium oxalate
   (b) Must consider in patients with pyelonephritis who remain febrile or have continued bacteriuria despite 48 h of antibiotics
   (c) Diagnose with US or MRI to limit radiation exposure to fetus *in utero*
   (d) Women with nephrolithiasis have a higher rate of preterm delivery
   (e) Most stones (70%) pass spontaneously. Others may need urologic intervention (i.e., ureteroscopy and stent placement)
      (i) YAG laser lithotripsy may be used in pregnancy; extracorporeal lithotripsy is not approved for use during pregnancy
   (f) Epidural may be used during conservative management of urolithiasis for pain relief (ureter sensory innervation is T11-L1)
      (i) Allows analgesia without systemic opioids, which impair normal ureteral peristalsis

Human Immunodeficiency Virus (HIV) Infection

46

1. Retrovirus (carries the enzyme reverse transcriptase) that has CNS involvement, long periods of clinical latency, and persistent viremia
2. Susceptible to bacterial, viral, fungal, parasitic, and mycobacterial infection and several malignancies (e.g., Kaposi's sarcoma, B-cell lymphoma, invasive cervical carcinoma)
3. Eventually affects multiple organ systems, but highly active antiretroviral therapy (HAART) makes it unlikely that pregnant patient will present with significant organ involvement
   (a) Neurologic
      (i) Early (initial infection): headache, photophobia, meningoencephalitis, cognitive and affective changes, cranial neuropathy, and peripheral neuropathy
      (ii) Latent phase: demyelinating neuropathy and CSF abnormalities
      (iii) Late (clinical AIDS): meningitis, focal brain lesions, diffuse encephalopathy, myelopathy (segmental or diffuse), peripheral neuropathy, and myopathy
   (b) Pulmonary
      (i) Due to opportunistic infections, mainly *P. carinii* pneumonia (PCP)
      (ii) Clinical picture is similar to ARDS (severe hypoxia and a pattern of diffuse interstitial infiltrates on CXR)
         1. Early corticosteroids decrease likelihood of progression to respiratory failure
         2. Survival puts patients at risk for pneumatoceles, which may rupture and cause pneumothorax
      (iii) Reactivation of latent Tb is common
   (c) Gastrointestinal
      (i) Painful or difficult swallowing due to herpetic, cytomegalovirus (CMV), or candida esophagitis

© Springer Nature Switzerland AG 2019
C. Wasson et al., *Absolute Obstetric Anesthesia Review*,
https://doi.org/10.1007/978-3-319-96980-0_46

    (ii) Severe diarrhea due to CMV, herpes simplex virus (HSV), *Shigella*, *Salmonella*, *Candida*, *Cryptosporidia*, *Giardia*, *Mycobacterium avium* complex (MAC), or HIV itself can lead to cachexia and electrolyte disturbances

    (iii) Hepatobiliary disease is common, including hepatitis B and C, CMV, mycobacterial infection (both *M. tuberculosis* and MAC), and *Cryptococcus*

(d) Hematologic

    (i) Leukopenia, especially depletion of CD4 lymphocytes

    (ii) Anemia

    (iii) Coagulation disturbances, including ITP

(e) Cardiovascular

    (i) Pericarditis usually due to mycobacterium

    (ii) Pulmonary HTN may develop due to episodes of PCP

    (iii) Clinical myocarditis or cardiomyopathy is rare

    (iv) Infective endocarditis due to IV drugs

(f) Endocrine

    (i) Abnormal thyroid function tests are common

    (ii) Insulin resistance and diabetes are consequences of HIV infection and antiretroviral treatment

(g) Renal

    (i) At risk for ARF due to sepsis, dehydration, and drug toxicity

    (ii) HIV-associated nephropathy is characterized by focal segmental glomerulosclerosis

4. Risk factors for vertical transmission of HIV: severity of maternal disease, maternal viral burden, viral genotype, sexually transmitted diseases (STDs), substance abuse, lack of maternal antiviral therapy, chorioamnionitis, prolonged ruptured membranes, invasive fetal monitoring, vaginal delivery, forceps delivery, breast feeding, and prematurity

5. HAART should be continued during pregnancy and is not teratogenic

    (a) In the absence of antiretroviral therapy, the risk of vertical transmission is ~25%

    (b) Risk reduces to 5–8% with treatment with zidovudine (ZDV)

    (c) The risk is ~2% if treated with ZDV and undergoes scheduled cesarean delivery

6. Women with viral load more than 1000 copies of viral RNA/ml should be counseled regarding the potential benefit of scheduled cesarean delivery to reduce the risk of vertical transmission.

7. Neuraxial anesthesia is safe in HIV-infected parturients.

8. High risk for having other STDs, including syphilis. Very important to perform a neurologic exam and document it prior to neuraxial anesthesia due to the neurologic effects of syphilis.

Part IV

Problems of Term and Delivery

Intrapartum Fetal Assessment

47

1. Fetal Heart Rate (FHR) Monitoring
   (a) Determines baseline rate and patterns of FHR in relationship to uterine contractions
   (b) Normal baseline FHR = 110–160 bpm
   (c) Decreased FHR variability is due to fetal hypoxia, fetal sleep state, fetal neurologic abnormality, and decreased CNS activity that results from exposure to drugs (e.g. opioids)
   (d) Early decelerations are from reflex vagal activity due to mild hypoxia or fetal head compression
   (e) Late decelerations are due to fetal hypoxemia secondary to uteroplacental insufficiency, decompensation of myocardial circulation, and myocardial failure
   (f) Variable decelerations are due to baroreceptor- or chemoreceptor-mediated vagal activity, usually from umbilical cord occlusion (either partial or complete)
   (g) Fetal movement causes FHR accelerations and indicate fetal health
2. Fetal scalp blood gases
   (a) An older method used to confirm or exclude the presence of fetal acidosis when FHR monitoring suggests fetal compromise
   (b) Indicated in decreased or absent FHR variability or persistent late or variable FHR decelerations.
   (c) Relative contraindications: presence of intact membranes and an unengaged vertex presentation; fetal coagulopathy (due to possible fetal exsanguination); infection (e.g. chorioamnionitis, HIV, or HSV); anticipated need for many samples
   (d) Fetal scalp blood pH > 7.25 is acceptable and labor may continue; pH < 7.20 is abnormal and delivery should be expedited; pH between 7.20 and 7.25 is indeterminent and should be repeated

© Springer Nature Switzerland AG 2019
C. Wasson et al., *Absolute Obstetric Anesthesia Review*,
https://doi.org/10.1007/978-3-319-96980-0_47

3. Fetal pulse ox
   (a) Used in term, singleton fetus <36 weeks gestation with vertex presentation and non-reassuring FHR pattern after rupture of membranes
   (b) Normal fetal SaO_2 is 35–65%

Supine Hypotensive Syndrome

48

1. Bradycardia and drop in BP with supination seen during normal pregnancy
2. Due to compression of the aorta and inferior vena cava by the gravid uterus
3. Signs/symptoms: pallor, tachycardia, sweating, nausea, hypotension, dizziness
4. All pregnant women over 20 weeks' gestation should be positioned with left uterine displacement to minimize aortocaval compression

© Springer Nature Switzerland AG 2019
C. Wasson et al., *Absolute Obstetric Anesthesia Review*,
https://doi.org/10.1007/978-3-319-96980-0_48

Embolic Disorders

49

1. Thromboembolism
   (a) Most often due to DVT, but may also occur due to superficial vein, puerperal septic pelvic vein, and puerperal ovarian vein thrombosis
   (b) Higher frequency of thromboembolism during pregnancy is attributed to Virchow's triad:
      (i) Increased venous stasis due to venocaval compression and decreased mobility
      (ii) Hypercoagulability of pregnancy (see discussion under hematology)
      (iii) Vascular injury (separation of placenta from uterine wall traumatizes the endometrium)
   (c) The highest risk for thromboembolic events is during the first postpartum week
      (i) Cesarean delivery doubles the risk for postpartum VTE compared to vaginal delivery
      (ii) Unplanned cesarean delivery has greater risk than elective cesarean delivery
   (d) Preeclampsia, multiple gestation, history of previous thromboembolism, and certain diseases (e.g., heart disease, smoking, obesity, antiphospholipid antibody syndrome, and thrombophilias (i.e., protein S and C deficiencies, antithrombin III deficiency, hyperhomocysteinemia, and prothrombin gene or factor V Leiden mutation)) increases risk
   (e) Manifestations and prognosis depend on: size/number of emboli, concurrent cardiopulmonary function, rate of clot fragmentation and lysis, presence or absence of a source for recurrent emboli, and location of the embolism (proximal or main pulmonary artery embolism is more symptomatic than segmental embolization)
   (f) Patient may complain of dyspnea, palpitations, anxiety, and chest pain

© Springer Nature Switzerland AG 2019
C. Wasson et al., *Absolute Obstetric Anesthesia Review*,
https://doi.org/10.1007/978-3-319-96980-0_49

(g) Physical exam suggestive of PE and % of patients affected: tachypnea (85%), localized rales (60%), accentuated second heart sound (50%), fever (45%), tachycardia (40%), thrombophlebitis (40%), supraventricular dysrhythmia (15%)

   (i) Signs of right ventricular failure (accentuated or split S2, jugular vein distention (JVD), parasternal heave, and hepatic enlargement) may be seen

   (ii) EKG may show right ventricular strain (right-axis deviation, P pulmonale, ST-T changes, T-wave inversion, supraventricular arrhythmias)

(h) Diagnosis:

   (i) D-dimer is elevated in normal pregnancy, so is non-specific

   (ii) PaO_2 can be normal in patients with PE (e.g., a normal PaO_2 does not exclude PE)

   (iii) If lower extremity US is positive with high clinical suspicion of PE, treatment is initiated

   (iv) If US is negative, CXR is performed

      1. If CXR is negative V:Q scan is performed

         (a) If V:Q is positive, treatment started

      2. If CXR is positive, CTA is performed

         (a) If CTA is positive, treatment started

(i) Unfractionated heparin is initiated immediately following the diagnosis of DVT for at least 5–7 days, after which SQ heparin can be substituted

   (i) Warfarin may be started after delivery and continued for at least 6 weeks postpartum

   (ii) Neuraxial anesthesia needs at least 12 h since the time of the last prophylactic dose of low molecular weight heparin; 24 h is needed for therapeutic doses

   (iii) Standard unfractionated heparin may be substituted for low molecular weight heparin near term to allow for aPTT monitoring. aPTT needs to be <40 s for neuraxial anesthesia to be instituted.

   (iv) Post-partum thromboprophylaxis with once daily LMWH needs 6–8 h after spinal or epidural placement prior to first dose; twice-daily dosing requires 24 h to elapse prior to first dose

   (v) Epidural catheter should be removed at least 10–12 h after the last dose of LMWH and the next dose should not be given sooner than 4 h after catheter removal

2. Amniotic fluid embolism (AFE)

  (a) Etiology is unclear

  (b) Biphasic response to AFE

   (i) Early phases is transient pulmonary vasospasm, likely from release of vasoactive substances. Vasospasm may account for the often fatal right heart dysfunction

   (ii) Second phase consists of left ventricular failure and pulmonary edema.

(c) Signs and symptoms: hypotension, fetal compromise, pulmonary edema or ARDS, cardiopulmonary arrest, cyanosis, seizure, atony, coagulopathy, dyspnea, bronchospasm, transient HTN, cough, headache, chest pain.

(d) Diagnosis of exclusion

    (i) Differential diagnosis: other obstetric complications (e.g., placental abruption, eclampsia); nonobstetric complications (e.g., PE, VAE, septic shock, MI, anaphylaxis); and anesthetic complications (e.g., total spinal anesthesia, systemic local anesthetic toxicity)

(e) Treatment is supportive

3. Venous air embolism (VAE)

(a) May account for transient symptoms (e.g., dyspnea, chest pain) and signs (e.g., sudden decrease in SaO_2, hypotension, arrhythmias) commonly encountered during cesarean

(b) Large volumes of air (>3 mL/kg) are fatal; smaller amounts can result in V:Q mismatch, hypoxemia, right heart failure, arrhythmias, and hypotension

(c) TEE is the most sensitive way to detect venous air embolism as low as 0.02 mL/kg

(d) Massive VAE can manifest as a sudden hypotension, hypoxemia, and even cardiac arrest.

    (i) Typically presents with chest pain, decreased SaO_2, and dyspnea

(e) EKG changes, including ST segment depression, are seen in 25–50% of all patients undergoing cesarean; it is unclear if VAE is responsible for these changes

(f) Treatment:

    (i) Prevent further air entrainment (e.g., flood surgical field with saline, change position (e.g. lower surgical field relative to heart if tolerated))

    (ii) Discontinue nitrous oxide and give 100% oxygen

    (iii) Support ventilation if needed.

        1. Avoid Valsalva and PEEP (an increase in right atrial pressure may cause paradoxical embolism)

    (iv) Support circulation

    (v) If hemodynamically unstable, consider placement of central venous catheter to aspirate air

    (vi) Expedite delivery

    (vii) Hyperbaric oxygen may improve neurologic outcomes if instituted within 6 hours of intracerebral air embolism

1. Placenta previa – placenta implants in front of the fetal presenting part
   (a) Total placenta previa completely covers the cervical os
   (b) Partial placenta previa covers part, but not all, of the os
   (c) Marginal placenta previa lies close to, but does not cover, the os
   (d) Conditions associated with previa: multiparity, advanced maternal age, previous cesarean delivery or other uterine surgery, and previous placenta previa
   (e) Diagnosis: painless vaginal bleeding during the second or third trimester
   (f) Confirmed with ultrasound
   (g) Active labor, a mature fetus, or persistent bleeding prompt cesarean delivery
      (i) Cesarean delivery required unless placenta is >2 cm from internal cervical os
   (h) Fetus at risk of preterm delivery, asymmetric intrauterine growth restriction, and higher incidence of congenital anomalies
   (i) Anesthetic considerations
      (i) Patients are at increased risk for intraoperative blood loss, so need two large-bore IVs. Increased risk due to:
         1. Uterine incision may cut an anterior placenta
         2. Lower uterine segment implantation sites do not contract as well as a fundal implantation site
         3. Higher risk of placenta accreta
      (ii) Type and screen is required. Type and cross for 2 units PRBCs is preferred (4 units if patient is actively bleeding)
      (iii) GA has a lower post-op hematocrit than neuraxial
      (iv) RSI with GA is preferred for actively bleeding patients; ketamine and etomidate are preferred induction agents

2. Placental abruption: complete or partial separation of the placenta from the decidua basalis before delivery of the fetus
   (a) May have vaginal bleeding, or bleeding may be concealed behind the placenta
   (b) Risk factors: HTN, preeclampsia, advanced maternal age, multiparity, maternal or paternal tobacco use, cocaine use, trauma, PROM, chorioamnionitis, bleeding in early pregnancy, and history of previous abruption
   (c) Presentation: vaginal bleeding, uterine tenderness, and increased uterine activity
   (d) Complications: hemorrhagic shock, acute renal failure, coagulopathy, and fetal compromise or demise
   (e) Term fetus without evidence of compromise undergoes induction of labor
      (i) If the fetus is preterm without compromise and abruption is minimal, pregnancy is continued for fetal lung maturation
      (ii) If compromise is evident, imminent delivery is necessary
   (f) Patient undergoing induction of labor may receive an epidural if she has normal coagulation studies
   (g) GA is preferred for most cases of urgent cesarean
   (h) Higher risk for persistent hemorrhage from uterine atony or coagulopathy
      (i) Replace coagulation factors and use uterotonic agents
3. Uterine rupture
   (a) Causes: previous uterine surgery, trauma (indirect (blunt (e.g., seat belt injury), excessive manual fundal pressure, extension of cervical laceration) or direct (penetrating wound, intrauterine manipulation, forceps application and rotation, postpartum curettage, manual placental extraction, external version)), inappropriate use of oxytocin, grand multiparity, uterine anomaly, placenta percreta, tumors (trophoblastic disease, cervical carcinoma), fetal problems (macrosomia, malposition, anomaly)
   (b) Suspect when vaginal bleeding, hypotension, cessation of labor, and fetal compromise are present
      (i) Pain occurs in <10% of patients with rupture
      (ii) Non-reassuring FHR pattern is the most reliable sign
   (c) Treatment: uterine repair, arterial ligation, or hysterectomy
   (d) GA is often necessary, unless patient has a preexisting epidural
4. Vasa previa: velamentous insertion of the fetal vessels over the cervical os (i.e., the fetal vessels traverse the fetal membranes ahead of the fetal presenting part)
   (a) Very high fetal mortality (50–70%)
   (b) Suspect if painless vaginal bleeding occurs with rupture of membranes, especially if accompanied by FHR decelerations or fetal bradycardia
   (c) If seen by prenatal US, cesarean delivery at 36 weeks' gestation
   (d) Ruptured vasa previa is a true emergency that requires immediate delivery of the fetus

Postpartum Hemorrhage

51

1. Hemorrhage is the leading cause of maternal mortality worldwide
2. Risk factors for peripartum hemorrhage: abnormal placentation, advanced maternal age, anticoagulation, bleeding disorder, chorioamnionitis, fetal demise, fetal malpresentation, GA, increased parity/grand multiparity, instrumental vaginal delivery, internal trauma (e.g., curettage, internal version), oxytocin augmentation of labor, placental abruption, precipitous delivery, preeclampsia (coagulopathy, thrombocytopenia), PROM, previous uterine surgery (cesarean delivery, myomectomy), prolonged labor, retained placenta, tocolytic therapy, trauma (blunt or penetrating), uterine distention (macrosomia, multiple gestation, polyhydramnios), uterine leiomyoma
3. Preparation for OB hemorrhage:
   (a) Review history for anemia or risk factors for hemorrhage
   (b) Consult with the OB team regarding presence of additional risk factors
   (c) Review reports of US or MRI of placentation
   (d) Obtain a blood sample for T&S or cross-match
   (e) Contact the blood bank to check blood availability
      (i) In certain high-risk cases (e.g., suspected placenta accreta), blood products should be physically present in the OR prior to surgical incision
   (f) Obtain and check necessary equipment (e.g., hotline) and establish large-bore IV access
4. Initial treatment
   (a) Management options
      (i) Volume resuscitate
      (ii) Order CBC and coagulation studies
      (iii) Prepare for hysterectomy
      (iv) Determine etiology: uterine atony; retained products of conception; lacerations, tears, uterine rupture; placenta accreta; coagulopathy

© Springer Nature Switzerland AG 2019
C. Wasson et al., *Absolute Obstetric Anesthesia Review*,
https://doi.org/10.1007/978-3-319-96980-0_51

(b) Invasive treatment options – performed when conservative measures fail to control bleeding

   (i) Uterine compression sutures may preserve fertility, but have a failure rate up to 30%

   (ii) Angiographic arterial embolization is used in coagulopathic patients.
      1. The vessels responsible for bleeding are embolized with Gelfoam, which provides a temporary occlusion.
      2. Blood flow slowly returns through the vessels
      3. Uterus and fertility are preserved.
      4. Success rate is 85–95%.
      5. Requires interventional radiologist.

   (iii) Uterine, ovarian, and internal iliac artery ligation is useful when other measures have failed.
      1. When successful, fertility is preserved
      2. Lower extremity ischemia and neuropathy have been reported
      3. Success rate of 85%

   (iv) Intrauterine balloon tamponade
      1. Success rate of 80%
      2. Preserves fertility

   (v) Hysterectomy – often the definitive treatment for postpartum hemorrhage
      1. Two most common indications: uterine atony and placenta accreta
      2. Increased blood loss during cesarean or postpartum hysterectomy compared to elective
         (a) EBL in emergency obstetric hysterectomy: 2526 mL
         (b) EBL in elective obstetric hysterectomy: 1319 mL
      3. 61% have complications: cardiac arrest, DIC, pulmonary edema, sepsis, or bladder injury

5. Uterine atony – most common cause of severe postpartum hemorrhage
   (a) Many cases are due to overdistention of the uterus
   (b) Causes: multiple gestation, macrosomia, polyhydramnios, high parity, prolonged labor, chorioamnionitis, precipitous labor, augmented labor, tocolytic agents, high concentration of a volatile anesthetic
   (c) Diagnosed by a soft postpartum uterus with vaginal bleeding
   (d) Treatment: Uterotonic drugs (i.e., IV oxytocin, Hemabate, Methergine, Cytotec), uterine massage, bimanual compression
      (i) Small percentage require transfusion, minimally invasive treatment options, or hysterectomy
      (ii) Administration of additional uterotonic agents may avoid need for hysterectomy
      (iii) If hemorrhage and atony persist despite uterotonic drugs, invasive techniques (e.g., embolization of uterine arteries, surgical ligation of arteries, and hysterectomy) must be considered

6. Genital trauma: most common childbirth injuries are lacerations and hematomas of the perineum, vagina, and cervix
   (a) Suspect in vaginal bleeding with a firm, contracted uterus
   (b) Vaginal hematoma is due to soft tissue injury during delivery or bleeding from the descending branch of the uterine artery
      (i) Risk factors: forceps, vacuum extraction, nulliparity, advanced maternal age, high birth weight, prolonged second stage of labor, multiple gestation, preeclampsia, and vulvovaginal varicosities
   (c) Vulvar hematoma involves branches of the pudendal artery
   (d) Treatment of small hematomas that are not enlarging is with ice packs and oral analgesics. Large hematomas need I&D
   (e) Retroperitoneal hematomas are uncommon, but dangerous
      (i) Due to laceration of branches of the hypogastric artery
      (ii) Usually occurs during cesarean or rarely after rupture of a low transverse uterine scar during labor
      (iii) Self-limiting retroperitoneal hematomas do not need surgical intervention. Life-threatening hematomas require exploratory laparotomy and ligation of the hypogastric vessels
7. Retained placenta: failure to deliver the placenta completely following delivery of the infant
   (a) Includes retained placental fragments
   (b) During early postpartum period, manual removal and inspection of the placenta may occur
   (c) If the obstetrician requests uterine relaxation to facilitate manual removal of the placenta, GA with volatiles will cause uterine relaxation, or, more commonly, administration of nitroglycerin
8. Placenta accreta: abnormally adherent placenta
   (a) Three types:
      (i) Placenta accreta: adherence to the myometrium without invasion of (or passage through) uterine muscle
      (ii) Placenta increta: invasion of the myometrium
      (iii) Placenta percreta: invasion of the uterine serosa or other pelvic structures
   (b) High risk in patients with a placenta previa or low-lying placenta with a history of previous cesarean delivery
   (c) Most patients require hysterectomy
   (d) Blood and clotting factors should be available for these patients as there is a high risk of hemorrhage
9. Uterine inversion: turning inside-out of all or part of the uterus
   (a) Risk factors: uterine atony, inappropriate fundal pressure, excessive umbilical cord traction, a short umbilical cord, and uterine anomalies
   (b) Treatment: prompt correction, possibly necessitating anesthesia for uterine relaxation (GA vs. nitroglycerin)

Cord Prolapse

52

1. Causes cord compression and subsequent sudden fetal bradycardia
2. Treatment is usually manual elevation of the fetal head and emergency cesarean delivery
3. Rarely, the umbilical cord is returned into the uterus and vaginal delivery attempted

© Springer Nature Switzerland AG 2019
C. Wasson et al., *Absolute Obstetric Anesthesia Review*,
https://doi.org/10.1007/978-3-319-96980-0_52

Dystocia, Malposition, and Malpresentation (Breech, Transverse Lie)

53

1. Shoulder dystocia
   (a) Anterior shoulder becomes trapped above the pubic symphysis
   (b) Umbilical cord compression, resulting in asphyxia, may occur if delivery is not accomplished quickly
   (c) Excessive traction on the fetal head may lead to brachial plexus injury (e.g., Erb's palsy), which may be permanent or temporary
   (d) Risk factors: maternal diabetes, fetal macrosomia, delayed active phase of labor, prolonged second stage of labor, operative vaginal delivery
   (e) Management:
       (i) Suprapubic pressure to dislodge the anterior shoulder from above the pubic symphysis
       (ii) Hyperflexion of maternal thighs beside abdomen (McRoberts maneuver) to rotate the pubic symphysis
       (iii) Intravaginal pressure on posterior shoulder to transform anterior-posterior shoulder position to oblique position
       (iv) Delivery of posterior arm to allow more room for delivery
       (v) Cephalic replacement (Zavanelli maneuver) to allow cesarean delivery
2. Malposition
   (a) Occiput posterior position may lead to prolonged labor that is associated with increased maternal discomfort
   (b) Vertex may remain occiput transverse
3. Malpresentation
   (a) Breech: fetal buttocks and/or lower extremities overlie the pelvic inlet
       (i) Frank breech: lower extremities flexed at the hips and extended at the knees
       (ii) Complete breech: lower extremities flexed at both the hips and the knees

C. Wasson et al., *Absolute Obstetric Anesthesia Review*,
https://doi.org/10.1007/978-3-319-96980-0_53

    (iii) Incomplete breech: one or both of the lower extremities is extended at the hips

    (iv) Risk factors for breech presentation:

       1. Uterine distention or relaxation (multiparity, multiple gestation, hydramnios, macrosomia)

       2. Abnormalities of the uterus or pelvis (pelvic tumors, uterine anomalies, pelvic contracture)

       3. Abnormalities of the fetus (hydrocephalus, anencephaly)

       4. Obstetric complications (previous breech delivery, preterm gestation, oligohydramnios, cornual-fundal placenta, placenta previa)

    (v) Obstetric management: external cephalic version, cesarean delivery (most commonly) vs. vaginal breech delivery

    (vi) Benefits of neuraxial analgesia: pain relief; inhibition of early pushing; ability of the parturient to push during the second stage and spontaneously deliver the infant to the level of the umbilicus; a relaxed pelvic flood and perineum at delivery; and the option to convert to surgical epidural if needed for emergency cesarean

(b) Brow presentation typically requires cesarean delivery due to dystocia

(c) Face presentation may be delivered vaginally if the mentum rotates to an anterior position

(d) Shoulder presentation/transverse lie mandates cesarean delivery, unless successful external cephalic version or internal podalic version and total breech extraction of a second twin with a shoulder presentation

Maternal Cardiopulmonary Resuscitation

54

1. Major causes of cardiac arrest during pregnancy: AFE, hemorrhage (DIC, placental abruption, placenta previa, uterine atony), iatrogenic (anesthetic complications, hypermagnesemia, medication errors or allergy), preexisting heart disease (congenital or acquired), pregnanc-induced HTN, sepsis, trauma, PE
2. If prior to delivery, left uterine displacement must be maintained and aortocaval compression avoided during resuscitation
3. ABCs as in non-pregnant (airway, ventilation, circulation)
   (a) The 2015 American Heart Association guideline recommends the same hand position for Chest compressions in pregnant women and nonpregnant adults. Manual uterine displacement during CPR to avoid aortocaval compression, optimize venous return, and generate adequate stroke volume
4. Standard cardiopulmonary resuscitation algorithms and pharmacologic therapy without modification
5. If resuscitative efforts are unsuccessful, emergency hysterotomy (perimortem cesarean) must be initiated at four minutes postarrest as it may be impossible to resuscitate the mother until adequate venous return is restored
   (a) Decision for delivery depends on gestational age, features of cardiac arrest (e.g. duration of arrest and hypoxemia) and professional setting (skills of surgeon, anesthesia provider, neonatologist, and presence of support personnel)
      (i) <20 weeks gestation, hysterotomy performed for maternal resuscitation, but fetus not viable
      (ii) >24 weeks, delivery improves chances of survival for both mother and baby
      (iii) Best infant survival when delivery occurs within 5 min of maternal arrest

© Springer Nature Switzerland AG 2019
C. Wasson et al., *Absolute Obstetric Anesthesia Review*,
https://doi.org/10.1007/978-3-319-96980-0_54

Fever and Infection

55

1. Fever: temperature >38°C
   (a) Increased body temperature causes vasodilation. If it is not adequate to prevent hyperthermia, sweating occurs for evaporative heat loss
   (b) Abnormal body temperature may occur from drugs or diseases, but is often due to infectious process of fetal membranes, urinary tract, respiratory tract, and postpartum uterine cavity
   (c) One-minute Apgar scores less than 7 and hypotonia are more common in babies of febrile mothers
   (d) Maternal fever may correlate with neonatal brain injury
2. Infection
   (a) Maternal-fetal infection has higher perinatal morbidity
   (b) Chorioamnionitis
      (i) Diagnosed based on signs (temp > 38.0 °C and maternal or fetal tachycardia, uterine tenderness, and/or foul-smelling amniotic fluid)
      (ii) Often polymicrobial and due to normal genital bacteria (e.g., *Bacteroides*, group B strep, and *E. coli*)
      (iii) Maternal complications: preterm labor, placental abruption, postpartum infection, uterine atony, postpartum hemorrhage, sepsis, and death
      (iv) Neonatal complications: pneumonia, meningitis, sepsis, and death
      (v) Strong correlation with cerebral palsy
      (vi) Early, antepartum antibiotic therapy decreases maternal and neonatal morbidity
   (c) Urologic infections
      (i) Urinary tract infection (UTI) is common during pregnancy. Asymptomatic UTI will ascend into the kidney and cause pyelonephritis
      (ii) Most common organisms: *E. coli*, *Klebsiella*, and *Proteus*
      (iii) Pyelonephritis may cause preterm labor and delivery
      (iv) Research supports screening and treating pregnant women for asymptomatic bacteriuria

© Springer Nature Switzerland AG 2019
C. Wasson et al., *Absolute Obstetric Anesthesia Review*,
https://doi.org/10.1007/978-3-319-96980-0_55

    (d) Respiratory tract infections
       (i) Most are viral upper respiratory infections (URIs)
      (ii) Infection often leads to maternal hypoxemia due to increased O_2 consumption and lower FRC
     (iii) Community-acquired pneumonias may occur
         1. Organisms: *S. pneumoniae* (most common), *Mycoplasma pneumonia*, and influenza
    (e) Postpartum infection
       (i) Most common source is genital tract
      (ii) Postpartum uterine infection symptoms: fever, malaise, abdominal pain, and purulent lochia
         1. More common post-cesarean than vaginal
    (f) Sepsis and septic shock – sepsis is rare and is a continuum
       (i) Systemic inflammatory response syndrome – two or more of the following signs: fever, leukocytosis, tachycardia, tachypnea
      (ii) Severe sepsis involves organ failure of at least one system
     (iii) Septic shock is hypotension and multiorgan hypoperfusion and failure
         1. Typically gram-negative bacteremia in pregnant women
         2. Usually due to untreated chorioamnionitis, pyelonephritis, endometritis, wound infection, incomplete abortion, and self-inducted abortion
         3. Rarely due to amniocentesis, medical abortion, dental procedures, and assisted reproductive technology
3. Epidural analgesia and maternal fever
    (a) Epidurals typically cause vasodilation and hypothermia
    (b) Neuraxial analgesia may cause a rise in temperature
       (i) Temperatures are unaffected for the first 4 h
      (ii) After 5 h, maternal temperatures may rise approximately 0.1 °C/h without signs of infection
     (iii) Mechanism unknown
         1. Thermoregulatory factors may play a role (e.g., ambient temperature, impaired heat dissipation, and increased heat production)
         2. Effect of systemic opioids in patients not receiving epidural analgesia may suppress fever that may have otherwise been apparent
         3. Inflammation
4. Neuraxial anesthesia in the febrile patient
    (a) No studies clearly established a causal relationship between dural puncture during bacteremia and the subsequent development of meningitis or epidural abscess
    (b) Meningitis after spinal anesthesia is likely from external contamination (of equipment) rather than blood-borne pathogens

   (c) Studies suggest meningitis and epidural abscess are very rare complications of epidural or spinal anesthesia

   (d) Bacteremia itself does not increase the risk of CNS infection after neuraxial anesthesia

   (e) High-grade bacteremia may increase the risk of meningitis after dural puncture, but antibiotic therapy before dural puncture reduces/eliminates the risk

   (f) Many anesthesiologists will administer neuraxial anesthesia to patients with systemic infection if appropriate antibiotic therapy has begun

1. Definition: labor (regular uterine contractions accompanied by change in cervical dilation to at least 2 cm) prior to 37 weeks' gestation.
2. Less than 10% of women with preterm labor give birth within 7 days of presentation.
3. Risk factors: demographic characteristics (non-white race, extremes of age (<17 or >35), low socioeconomic status, low prepregnancy body mass index (BMI), history of preterm delivery, interpregnancy interval <6 months, abnormal uterine anatomy (myomas), abnormal cervical anatomy, trauma, abdominal surgery during pregnancy, acute or chronic systemic disease), behavioral factors (physically strenuous work, psychological stress, tobacco use, substance abuse), obstetric factors (vaginal bleeding, infection (systemic, genital tract, periodontal), cervical length/incompetent cervix, multiple gestation, assisted reproductive technologies, preterm PROM, abnormal fetal placentation, polyhydramnios), and fetal factors (genetic abnormalities and fetal death)
4. Infection is thought to be present in up to 40% of preterm deliveries
    (a) Often due to untreated acute pyelonephritis
    (b) Other commonly identified organisms: *Ureaplasma urealyticum*, *Bacteroides* species, *N. gonorrhoeae*, *C. trachomatis*, group B streptococcus (GBS), *S. aureus*, *T. pallidum*, and enteropharyngeal bacteria
5. Several methods to predict preterm birth have been proposed:
    (a) Home uterine activity monitoring – insufficient data to support benefit in preventing preterm birth
    (b) Salivary estriol measurement – surge in maternal estriol levels occurs approximately 3 weeks prior to delivery. Specificity of test is too low for the test to be clinically useful
    (c) Screening for bacterial vaginosis – bacterial vaginosis is associated with an increased risk of preterm delivery
    (d) Fetal fibronectin screening – a positive test at 22–24 weeks' gestation is 63% sensitive in predicting preterm labor before 28 weeks' gestation. If test is negative, risk of preterm delivery within 1 or 2 weeks is <1%

© Springer Nature Switzerland AG 2019
C. Wasson et al., *Absolute Obstetric Anesthesia Review*,
https://doi.org/10.1007/978-3-319-96980-0_56

(e) Cervical ultrasonography – short cervical length is associated with increased risk of preterm labor.

(f) Interventions to prevent preterm labor and delivery (most have not been shown to alter outcome): suppression of uterine contractions; antimicrobial therapy; prophylactic cervical cerclage; maternal nutritional supplements; reduction in maternal stress; and hormonal therapy

6. Short course of tocolytic therapy may delay delivery for 24–48 h (enough to transfer to a facility that can provide care for the preterm neonate, administer a corticosteroid to accelerate fetal lung maturity, and administer antibiotics to prevent neonatal GBS infection)

(a) ACOG discourages the prolonged use of tocolysis after corticosteroid administration is complete (usually 48 h)

7. Contraindications to tocolytics for preterm labor: fetal death, fetal anomalies incompatible with life, nonreassuring fetal status, chorioamnionitis/fever of unknown origin, severe hemorrhage, and severe chronic and/or pregnancy-induced HTN

8. Specific tocolytic drugs:

(a) Calcium channel blockers

    (i) Contraindications: cardiac disease, renal disease, maternal hypotension, concomitant magnesium therapy

    (ii) Maternal side effects: transient hypotension, flushing, headache, dizziness, nausea

    (iii) Fetal side effects: none

(b) Cyclooxygenase inhibitors (NSAIDs)

    (i) Contraindications: significant renal or hepatic impairment, active peptic ulcer disease, coagulation disorders or thrombocytopenia, NSAID-sensitive asthma, other NSAID sensitivities

    (ii) Maternal side effects: nausea, heartburn

    (iii) Fetal/neonatal side effects: constriction of the ductus arteriosus, pulmonary hypertension, reversible renal dysfunction (leading to oligohydramnios), intraventricular hemorrhage (IVH), hyperbilirubinemia, necrotizing enterocolitis

(c) Beta-agonists

    (i) Contraindications: cardiac dysrhythmias, poorly controlled thyroid disease, poorly controlled DM

    (ii) Maternal side effects: cardiopulmonary (dysrhythmias, pulmonary edema, myocardial ischemia, hypotension, tachycardia), metabolic (hyperglycemia, hyperinsulinemia, hypokalemia, antidiuresis, altered thyroid function), other (tremor, palpitations, nervousness, nausea/vomiting, fever, hallucinations)

    (iii) Fetal side effects: tachycardia, hyperinsulinemia, hyperglycemia, myocardial and septal hypertrophy, myocardial ischemia

    (iv) Neonatal side effects: tachycardia, hypoglycemia, hypocalcemia, hyperbilirubinemia, hypotension, IVH

   (d) Magnesium sulfate
- (i) Also used as neuroprotection in anticipated early preterm delivery (i.e., 24–32 weeks' gestation) to decrease the risk of cerebral palsy in surviving infants
- (ii) Contraindications: myasthenia gravis, myotonic dystrophy
- (iii) Maternal side effects: flushing, lethargy, headache, muscle weakness, diplopia, dry mouth, pulmonary edema, cardiac arrest
- (iv) Fetal/neonatal side effects: lethargy, hypotonia, respiratory depression, demineralization (prolonged use)

9. Neuraxial analgesia during vaginal delivery of the preterm infant lead to:
   - (a) Inhibition of inappropriate maternal expulsive efforts before complete cervical dilation, especially in breech presentation
   - (b) Prevention of precipitous delivery, which can cause rapid decompression of the infant's head and increased risk of intracranial hemorrhage
   - (c) Provision of a relaxed pelvic floor and perineum to facilitate a smooth, controlled delivery of the preterm infant's head

Vaginal Birth After Cesarean Section (VBAC)

57

1. A Classic uterine incision is high risk for catastrophic uterine rupture during a subsequent pregnancy (both before or during labor) and increases maternal and perinatal morbidity or mortality
2. Low-transverse uterine incision has less blood loss and better healing, with better maintenance of integrity in subsequent pregnancies
3. Trial of labor is successful in 60–80% of women
4. Previous successful vaginal delivery is the greatest predictor for successful VBAC
5. History of dystocia, a need for induction of labor, and maternal obesity are associated with a lower likelihood of successful VBAC
6. Contraindications for VBAC:
   (a) Previous classic or T-shaped incision or extensive transfundal uterine surgery
   (b) Previous uterine rupture
   (c) Medical or obstetric complication that precludes vaginal delivery
   (d) Inability to perform emergency cesarean delivery because of unavailable surgeon, anesthesia (provider), sufficient staff or facility
   (e) Two prior uterine scars and no vaginal deliveries
7. All VBAC patients should be type-and-crossed
8. Epidural analgesia does not delay the diagnosis of uterine rupture or decrease the likelihood of successful VBAC

C. Wasson et al., *Absolute Obstetric Anesthesia Review*,
https://doi.org/10.1007/978-3-319-96980-0_57

Multiple Gestation

58

1. Exaggerated cardiovascular and pulmonary changes of pregnancy
2. Increased risk of uterine atony and postpartum hemorrhage due to greater uterine distention, necessitating large-bore IV access prior to delivery
3. Increased risk of aortocaval compression and hypotension
4. Greater O_2 consumption and decreased FRC compared to singleton pregnancies

© Springer Nature Switzerland AG 2019
C. Wasson et al., *Absolute Obstetric Anesthesia Review*,
https://doi.org/10.1007/978-3-319-96980-0_58

Resuscitation of Newborn

59

1. Apgar scoring
   (a) Scoring system to help differentiate infants who require resuscitation from those who need routine care. Apgar score should not be used to predict neonatal mortality or morbidity as it is not an accurate prognostic tool for these outcomes
   (b) Five parameters that are assessed at 1 and 5 min after birth and receive scores of 0, 1, or 2
   (c) Table 59.1: APGAR scoring
   (d) Score 8–10 is normal; 4–7 indicates moderate impairment; 0–3 signals need for immediate resuscitation

2. Umbilical Cord Blood Gas Measurements
   (a) Reflect the fetal condition immediately before delivery and are more objective than Apgar score
   (b) ACOG recommends cord blood gas for cesarean delivery for fetal compromise, low 5-min Apgar score, severe growth restriction, abnormal FHR tracing, maternal thyroid disease, intrapartum fever, and/or multiple gestation

Table 59.1 Apgar Scoring System. The score is universally used to assess the status of the newborn infant immediately at 1 and 5 minutes of age

Parameter	0	1	2
Color	Cyanotic	Acrocyanotic (trunk pink, extremities blue)	Pink
Respiratory effort	Absent	Irregular, slow, shallow, or gasping	Robust, crying
Heart rate	Absent	<100	>100
Reflex irritability (nasal catheter, oropharyngeal suctioning)	No response	Grimace	Active coughing and sneezing
Muscle Tone	Absent, limp	Some flexion of extremities	Active movement

© Springer Nature Switzerland AG 2019
C. Wasson et al., *Absolute Obstetric Anesthesia Review*,
https://doi.org/10.1007/978-3-319-96980-0_59

   (c) Umbilical artery blood gas reflects fetal condition
   (d) Umbilical vein is maternal condition and uteroplacental gas exchange
3. Techniques and Pharmacology of Resuscitation
   (a) Mouth and then nose is suctioned as soon as head is delivered (prior to first breath) to remove residual amniotic fluid, mucus, blood, and meconium
   (b) Neonatal table should be adjustable to allow for 30° Trendelenburg (favors drainage of secretions) and reverse Trendelenburg (may increase PaO_2 during spontaneous ventilation)
   (c) Place neonate in warm, dry blanket promptly (hypothermia can cause greater O_2 consumption, metabolic acidosis, and higher mortality rate)
   (d) Tactile stimulation if newborn does not breathe immediately
       (i) If ventilation not stimulated, begin positive-pressure mask ventilation
   (e) First sign of adequate ventilation is an increase in heart rate; color change occurs slowly
   (f) Positive-pressure ventilation can be stopped when HR > 100 bpm
   (g) Majority of neonates do not need chest compressions or medications as they respond to ventilatory support.
   (h) Chest compressions are indicated when HR < 60 bpm despite adequate ventilation with supplemental O_2 for 30 s
   (i) Epinephrine (0.01–0.03 mg/kg or 0.1–0.3 mL/kg of a 1:10,000 solution) is the drug recommended for use during neonatal resuscitation
       (i) Administer if HR remains <60 bpm after 30 s of adequate ventilation and chest compressions
   (j) Calcium, bicarb, and atropine are not recommended.
   (k) Volume expanders should be considered when the newborn demonstrates signs of shock (pale skin, poor perfusion, weak pulse) or has not shown adequate response to resuscitative measures
       (i) NS or LR at 10 mL/kg over 5–10 min
       (ii) O-negative packed RBC if heavy blood loss is suspected

Intrauterine Surgery

60

1. Useful for certain correctable fetal anomalies with predictable, life-threatening, or serious developmental consequences, such as conditions that can interfere with fetal organ development or cause high-output cardiac failure
2. Examples:
   (a) Obstructive hydronephrosis – can lead to oligohydramnios and subsequent fetal pulmonary hypoplasia
   (b) Congenital diaphragmatic hernia – can cause fetal pulmonary hypoplasia
   (c) Congenital cystic adenomatoid malformation – pulmonary tumor with cystic and solid components and can cause hydrops fetalis, mediastinal shift, and pulmonary hypoplasia
   (d) Sacrococcygeal teratoma – functions as large AV fistulas that can lead to hydrops fetalis, placentomegaly, and intra-uterine fetal demise due to high-output cardiac failure or intra-uterine rupture and fetal hemorrhage
   (e) Myelomeningocele – can result in lifelong morbidity and disability, including paraplegia, incontinence, hydrocephalus, and impaired cognition
   (f) Twin-to-twin transfusion syndrome – increased mortality
      (i) Polycythemia, polyuria, polyhydramnios, and hypertrophic cardiomyopathy in recipient twin leading to hydrops fetalis and fetal death
      (ii) Hypovolemia, oliguria, growth-restriction, oligohydramnios in donor twin leading to renal failure
   (g) Twin reversed arterial perfusion sequence – one twin perfuses the second by retrograde flow through arterioarterial anastomoses
      (i) Causes high-output cardiac failure in the normal ("pump") twin with high mortality rate
      (ii) Perfused twin develops lethal anomalies, including acardia and acephalus
   (h) Congenital heart defects – ventricular outflow tract obstruction, aortic stenosis with developing hypoplastic left heart syndrome, pulmonary atresia without ventricular septal defect, and evolving hypoplastic right heart syndrome.

3. Not useful for nonlethal defects, such as craniofacial deformities
4. Maternal risks: blood loss, infection, placental abruption, and pulmonary edema due to tocolytic therapy (nitroglycerin)
5. Postop fetal complications: CNS injuries, postop amniotic fluid leaks, membrane separation, preterm PROM, preterm labor, and preterm delivery
6. Intrauterine fetal resuscitation – medications given IM or via umbilical artery
    (a) Atropine 0.02 mg/kg
    (b) Epinephrine 1 µg/kg
    (c) Crystalloid 10 mL/kg
    (d) O-negative, CMV-negative, leukocyte-depleted blood for fetal transfusion should be available if needed

Appendix A: Management of Antithrombotic Therapy for Neuraxial Procedures

Medication	Minimum time after last dose prior to neuraxial injection or catheter placement	Guidelines for use while neuraxial catheter is in place	Minimum time after neuraxial injection or catheter placement and next dose
Anticoagulants for VTE prophylaxis			
Unfractionated heparin 5000 units q8h or q12h	No time restrictions or contraindications		
Unfractionated heparin 7500 units SQ q8h	8 h	Contraindicated while catheter in place	4 h
Foundaparinux (Arixtra) 2.5 mg SQ daily	48 h (longer in renal impairment)		
Enoxaparin (Lovenox) 30 or 40 mg SQ q12h	12 h (longer in renal impairment)		
Enoxaparin (Lovenox) 40 mg SQ daily		Wait 8 h after catheter placement; wait 12 h after last dose before removing catheter	
Dalteparin (Fragmin) 5000 units SQ daily			
Apixaban (Eliquis) 2.5 mg BID	48 h (longer in renal impairment)		6 h
Rivaroxaban (Xarelto) 10 mg po daily			

© Springer Nature Switzerland AG 2019
C. Wasson et al., *Absolute Obstetric Anesthesia Review*,
https://doi.org/10.1007/978-3-319-96980-0

Medication	Minimum time after last dose prior to neuraxial injection or catheter placement	Guidelines for use while neuraxial catheter is in place	Minimum time after neuraxial injection or catheter placement and next dose
Agents for full systemic anticoagulation			
Dabigatran (Pradaxa) 75–150 mg BID	72 h (longer in renal impairment)	Contraindicated while catheter in place	6 h
Apixaban (Eliquis) 2.5–10 mg BID	48 h (longer in renal impairment)		
Edoxaban (Savaysa) 30–60 mg daily			
Rivaroxaban (Xarelto) 15–20 mg daily or 15 mg BID			
Dalteparin (Fragmin) 200 units/kg SQ daily or 100 units/kg SQ Q12h	24 h (longer in renal impairment)		4 h
Enoxaparin (Lovenox) 1.0–1.5 mg/kg SQ daily or 1 mg/kg SQ Q12h			
Fondaparinux (Arixtra) 5–10 mg SQ daily	72 h (longer in renal impairment)		
Unfractionated heparin IV infusion or full dose SQ	When aPTT <40 s		
Warfarin (Coumadin)	When INR <1.5		
Direct Thrombin Inhibitors, Injectable			
Argatroban IV continuous infusion	When DTI assay <40 or aPTT <40 s	Contraindicated while catheter in place	4 h
Bivalirudin (angiomax) IV continuous infusion			
Antiplatelet Agents			
Aspirin or NSAIDs	No time restrictions or contraindications		
Eptifibatide (integrelin)	8 h (longer in renal impairment)	Contraindicated while catheter in place	6 h
Tirofiban (Aggrestat)			
Abciximab (Reopro)	48 h		
Aspirin/dipyridamole (Aggrenox)	7 days		
Clopidogrel (Plavix)			
Prasugrel (Effient)			
Ticagrelor (Brillinta)			
Thrombolytic Agents			
Alteplase (TPA) 1mg dose for catheter clearance	No time restrictions or contraindications		
Alteplase (TPA) full dose for stroke, MI, etc	10 days	Contraindicated while catheter in place	10 days

Index

Printed in the United States
By Bookmasters